The Diet Docs
And The AMAZING
Metabolic Transformation

(dr.joe@thedietdoc.com)

All the information presented in this text is for educational and resource purposes only. It is there to help you make informed decisions about health related fitness issues. It is NOT a substitute for any advice given to you by your physician. Always consult your physician or health care provider before beginning any nutrition or exercise program. Use of the programs, advice, and information contained in this text is at the sole choice and risk of the reader. YOU are solely responsible for the way you perceive and utilize information in this text and you do so at your own risk. In no way will Joe Klemczewski or J. Scott Uloth or any persons and or entities associated with The Diet Docs, LLC be held responsible for any injuries or problems that may occur due to the use of this text or the advice contained therein. Prior to beginning any physical fitness regimen or making any nutritional changes you are strongly urged to consult your physician first.

The Diet Docs And The AMAZING Metabolic Transformation

Joe Klemczewski, Ph.D.

J. Scott Uloth, M.D.

Copyright © 2007 by Joe Klemczewski, Ph.D. and J. Scott Uloth, M.D..
The Diet Docs, LLC.

ISBN: Hardcover   978-1-4257-4846-3
            Softcover   978-1-4257-4845-6

All rights reserved. No part of this book may be reproduced or transmitted in any form or by any means, electronic or mechanical, including photocopying, recording, or by any information storage and retrieval system, without permission in writing from the copyright owner.

This book was printed in the United States of America.

To order additional copies of this book, contact:
Xlibris Corporation
1-888-795-4274
www.Xlibris.com
Orders@Xlibris.com
38305

CONTENTS

Introduction 9

Chapter One: Getting Started.. 17
Chapter Two: The Diet Docs' Rx... 30
Chapter Three: Meal Structuring—power Spacing............................. 46
Chapter Four: Carbohydrates: They're Not Just for Breakfast Anymore.....53
Chapter Five: The Skinny on Fat... 67
Chapter Six: Protein 78
Chapter Seven: Meal Ratios... 85
Chapter Eight: Recipes and Food Preparation 90
Chapter Nine: The Psychology of Success 140
Chapter Ten: Putting it All Together 157
Chapter Eleven: Six Weeks to Metabolic Transformation 160
Chapter Twelve: Pitfalls and Obstacles 172
Chapter Thirteen: The Health Benefits of Good Nutrition 186
Chapter Fourteen: Keep it Off Forever! 204

Epilogue: A Diet Doc—Three Years Later....................................... 207
Bibliography 209

DEDICATION

To my beautiful wife Gina who has been there through everything: I adore you and could never do what I do without your love and support. To Matthew, Grace, and Bethany: you are the best kids ever! I love you, and I am proud to be your daddy. To my family and my spectacular in-laws (the whole crew of you!), I thank you for always being there for me, looking out for me and encouraging me.

To our small groups, our church family and leadership at CFC, the entire crew at West Side Family Medicine, and to our patients and clients that have trusted us with their health, we are forever grateful and indebted.

And to our Lord and Savior, Jesus Christ, through You all things are possible. We praise You.

-Scott

Tracy, you give way more than you receive—the greatest soul-mate a guy could ever hope for. Though I sure don't deserve you, I wouldn't want a day without you. Cameron, Ashlyn, Trey, and Lynnea, I think you're going to change the world—you've certainly changed mine. What great young men and women you're becoming!

Mom and Dad, it all started with you. Thank you for teaching me how to work, Dad. Mom, thank you for showing me creativity and that I can achieve anything I can dream.

My clients, colleagues, and friends, you've taught me as much as I've taught you. Thank you for sharpening me and making the journey fun.

The ultimate thanks goes to my Father in Heaven for loving me even when I'm unlovable, Your Son—my Savior—for buying my eternity at the greatest cost, and Your Spirit for being faithful even when I'm not.

-Joe

The Diet Docs' Rx

- Document everything.
- Only one "splurge" meal per week (not a day or a weekend or…).
- Eat five to six times per day (three meals and two to three snacks).
- Eat even if you don't feel hungry initially to prevent bingeing ("stay ahead of hunger").
- Weigh/measure your food initially (make sure an ounce is an ounce, a cup is a cup…).
- Read labels carefully and watch portion size.
- Exercise five to six times per week and try to strength train at least two of those days.
- Keep constantly armed with good foods.

My Personal Rx (grams/day)

Protein _____

Carbs _____

Fat _____

INTRODUCTION

"Just how in the world did I get here?" The flashing red lights blinked between my toes as I asked that question over and over. Two hundred twenty-nine and a half pounds. I am the perfect weight if I were a 6'2" linebacker for the Colts. However, I am 5'8" (5'7 ¾" as my wife is quick to remind me), and I have the 40-yard dash speed of a 3-legged turtle. That last half-pound seems to taunt me, and I curse myself for buying a digital scale. I'm closing in on 40, and I am 60 to 70 pounds overweight. How in the heck did this happen?

I am sure this scene from my own life is repeated multiple times a day in the bathrooms or locker rooms across the United States: people staring at a scale and wondering how they went from the svelte, healthy kids of the past to the overweight, chronically sick and fatigued adults of the present. The blinking red numbers are the warning lights of our own impending doom. The next disaster film for the United States shouldn't feature a wayward comet, global warming, or icebergs, but our own swelling abdomens and poor health brought on by lack of proper nutrition, lack of exercise, and our woeful lack of information. ("Captain, the 32-ounce soda cup is about to crash into the Atlantic and give everyone on the Eastern seaboard diabetes! What shall we do?!") Scares me. Does it scare you? According to the PBS documentary *Diet Wars*, 50% of our nation's children will become afflicted with diabetes and all its complications. Obesity may soon replace smoking as the single largest preventable cause of death in the United States. In a country that prides itself on being the best, we are doing a darn good job of being the best at harming ourselves. Perhaps what we need to avert disaster is practical information that we can realistically incorporate into our daily lives. We need a weight-loss plan that is attainable and sustainable, a plan that provides flexibility within a framework.

My problems started almost immediately after high school. I believed that I needed sugar and caffeine to stay conscious in college, so Mr. Mountain Dew and I were tight. I used to drink so much soda that I once took two No-doz and fell asleep. No joke. The fact that I stopped running cross-country to focus on my studies helped expand my girth as well. Then there was the never-ending supply of fattening food at the student union hall where I would eat a bowl of Captain Crunch for dessert after a huge meal. My "freshman five" quickly turned into the "freshman fifteen." It deteriorated from there. I easily rationalized my behavior by believing that I was simply sacrificing my health in pursuit of knowledge, a good job, and helping others. Seemed like a decent trade at the time.

However, I always labored under the delusion of a former athlete that at any time I could "turn it on" and instantly return to the 155 pounds I was when I graduated high school. Needless to say, by my senior year of college, I had gained 40 pounds. As I was planning to marry my high school sweetheart, I started bike riding, lifting weights, and playing basketball. The fact that I had been accepted to medical school helped me to actively engage in those "non-academic pursuits" the entire second semester of my senior year. My dietary habits hadn't changed, but I eventually managed to work off 20 pounds and was down to 175 at my wedding. I was proud of myself, and didn't think I looked half bad. It didn't last.

Four years of medical school and three years of residency in family practice helped solidify my Mountain Dew addiction and my rationalizing skills. My education did help improve my knowledge of nutrition to a certain extent. It was the application part that gave me a bit of a problem. "Oh, I really don't feel that bad. So what if I have a stroke walking a flight of stairs or that my knees and arches hurt constantly? What's that? Oh, my blood pressure is up too? Well, just give me a pill or I'll grab something out of the sample medicine closet and I'll be fine." In our Lamaze class when the husbands had to wear the padded "sympathy belly" I joked that I didn't need one since I already looked nine months pregnant. Frankly, the number of people that patted my stomach and asked me when I was due was more than a little bit annoying. I knew that I would never shop in the "tall" section, but having to purchase suits in the "big" section was really bumming me out. I wish I could say that my nightmare on the scale was enough to stop me, but I simply quit weighing myself. Out of sight, out of mind. If I eat the ice cream with a spoon right out of the container and don't make the effort to get a bowl, those calories don't *really* count, do they?

How many of us delude ourselves into believing that we'll be "just fine"? How many of us don't go to our doctors because we are scared of what we might find? How many of us believe that we need to make a serious life change, but don't have the necessary information to succeed? How many of us live in fear that we can't do anything about it any way, no matter how hard we try? And how many of us are stuck in habits that we think we just can't break? ("Gotta have that soft drink in the morning or I just can't start my day.") I have news for you: I was right there with you, and I believed all of those lies. I thought I was simply doomed to be "fat and happy." Even though I had a doctorate-level education in medicine, I didn't have the information to help myself. I knew I needed assistance, and that's where this book comes in.

I am blessed to live in the same community as "Dr. Joe" and had witnessed the amazing transformation (the Metabolic Transformation) of several people who attended our church. These people were 20 years older than I, had lost weight, looked wonderful, and bragged about how great their energy was. So I bit my lip, sat on my ego, and was finally able to admit that I had a problem that I thought I was powerless over and that I needed help. Joe is one of the unique individuals who has spent a career combining academic learning with real-world education. He has a degree in physical therapy and two doctorates, including one in health and physical education. He's also a professional bodybuilder with arms that make him look like Popeye the trainer man. He knows what he is talking about. After a year and a half of working on my own, I felt I had conquered the exercise demon, walking on my treadmill regularly. However, I definitely needed more information about nutrition and the importance of weight lifting. I had only dropped from 230 to 213.5 when I arrived at Joe's doorstep. After consulting with him, I learned more about nutrition than I had learned in my first semester of medical school. He is truly the Sergeant Joe Friday of nutritionists. This book is the culmination of our knowledge (mainly 80% his and 20% mine or maybe 90/10—I'll have to think about it). It is "just the facts."

The key thing is that Joe and I are not just health or medical "gurus." We're just a couple of hard-working, regular Joes (well, one regular Joe and one slightly irregular Scott), who both continue to actively practice in our respective fields. We are not here to make this a nebulous affair where you come away feeling that you can't do anything without us. Our goal is for you to arrive at that moment of true understanding. That light bulb switching on in someone's head is what we strive for and what makes it all worthwhile. People are often swept away by the murkiness of the science of nutrition and throw their hands upward in disgust (the way I often do with my computer). However, nutrition is a "hard science" with testable end points. It is unfortunately clouded by all the psychological baggage that we attach to food. Heck, Dr. Phil has a whole book on that! But let me stress that this book will show you how to reach those end points in an easy-to-understand fashion. Some people want to be told "eat this" or "don't eat that," which this book can do to a point. But that won't forge a lasting change in behavior. Only with *understanding* do we develop a lifetime of healthy eating. We want to be your partners to help achieve that goal. There is no magic or voodoo necessary to make those unwanted inches around your middle go away. It's science but it ain't rocket science. With a few rare medical exceptions, there is absolutely no reason someone cannot lose weight if they diet properly and exercise. I wish I had a nickel for every person who came into my practice blaming a "thyroid disorder" for causing them to be overweight, only to sit there the next week with normal blood chemistry, facing the same questions about their obesity.

In this book, you will learn the value of your own personal "macronutrient range" (The Diet Docs' Rx). This critical range of macronutrients keeps you losing weight without making your body think it's starving, thus slowing down your metabolism. The Diet Docs' Rx chart provides the proper amounts of protein, carbohydrates, and fat for men and women based on height. You will learn how to glean nutritional information right from the label without having to use a calculator or a laptop. This information is readily available and not artificially contrived. You will learn to pay attention and not be fooled by portion sizes. People simply want to know what enough is, and after reading this text, you will finally know. As my eight-year-old Gracie says, "We're not on a diet; we're on a healthy eating plan!" This is a program that restricts calories by tailoring protein, carbohydrates, and fat to levels that fit your body structure and body type without over-utilizing any one of these nutrients. You will benefit from the clinical application of this diet that has helped others combat the conditions of diabetes, coronary artery disease, hyperlipidemia, and osteoarthritis. Finally, you will learn from someone who lost over 60 pounds what it was like and how you can do it as well. We will stress the themes of nutrition, exercise, discipline, and fun that lead to permanent weight loss and ultimately good health.

But we all must come to that moment of truth when we stop making excuses. I am a physician who works 60 to 80 hours per week. My day used to consist of arriving at the hospital by 7:00 a.m., doing rounds on my patients, then going to the office, seeing patients all day with 10 to 15 minutes for lunch, and being so busy I didn't even feel that I had time to go to the bathroom. (Is that bathroom comment too much information?) I would then get home between 6:30 and 7:00 p.m., eat dinner, play with my three children, help get them ready for bed, and start working on paperwork at 9:00 p.m. I would usually finish between 11:00 p.m. and 12:00 a.m. Rinse and repeat, day after day. I had developed extraordinary discipline in my business life, but chaos theory ruled my eating habits. "Anything, any time, anywhere" became my mantra. Maybe I just wanted some aspect of my life that I didn't have to care about, at least not now anyway. Maybe I just wanted to have fun. Food is fun, but it is also fuel and can't be viewed simply as a recreational activity. If you shoot 100 on the golf course, who cares unless you're Tiger Woods? If you're 100 pounds overweight, then that's a big deal!

When could I find time to exercise? When could I find the time to eat right? I had to be mentally sharp. I needed those three sodas a day. But don't cry for me, Argentina. I'm a big boy and I chose this life and how I was going to live or mis-live it. Then one day I realized that I could fall over dead and some people would simply step over my corpse and say, "Oh, poor Dr. Uloth. He was such a nice man. I wish he had taken better care of himself. I wonder who else in town is taking new patients." Doesn't matter what your job is or how important you think you might be. Game over, man. Game over.

No one else will do it for you. Not your mama, your daddy, or your spouse. You have to decide, like Morgan Freeman asked in *The Shawshank Redemption*, are you going to "get busy living or get busy dying?" I came to understand that as long as I was still vertical I wasn't going down without a fight, especially for the people that needed and loved me. I realized that God tells us to treat our bodies like a temple and mine was in utter disrepair. I had a tee shirt that said "God's property" on it, and one of my friends quipped, "Yeah, if that's God's property it ought to be condemned!" I realized that I was robbing my wife. I was setting a shameful example for my patients, and more importantly, my children. I realized that I wasn't going to be "just fine" unless I did something about it. I also realized that doctors exist to help prevent disease instead of just treating it. I always believed that principle about smoking, alcohol, drugs, cancer, but I allowed my weight to render me mute about the subject of obesity. Trust me: it's a darn sight better to be eating tuna on the outside of the hospital rather than sipping your dinner through a straw in the post-op recovery room. You need to be proactive for your own health. This is serious business folks, and this book is serious about showing you the path to a better life. That path, although narrow, is a lot more fun to run down with your family than to waddle down the wide path in agony. Dr. Joe and I believe that life is to be lived joyously, so we inject humor to keep your spirits up, but the end result of following this program is way powerful.

At the time of this writing, I have gone from 230 to 169.5 (44 pounds lost with Joe in 6 months as opposed to the 16 I lost in 18 months on my own). I am currently past the original goal of 172 that is a "healthy" weight for my height. Now, I'm glad I have a scale that weighs in half-pound intervals! I just bought a pair of 34" pants and took my 42's to the Salvation Army. I have run the first consecutive mile that I have run since high school. Do I have a "six-pack" yet? Nope and I probably never will, but I can see a little definition in my abs rather than my belly obscuring my toes when I look down. Instead of "abs of steel," I'll be happy with abs of aluminum foil. This book has given me the information that I need. In family practice, if you need a partner on a tough problem, you call in a specialist. Joe is that specialist. He helped me to understand that I didn't have to lose all that weight in 90 days or any other unrealistic time frame. He drove home the fact that it took years to build up and that it would take 6 to 12 months, or more, to get the weight off and to tone up muscles so that I would achieve the results I wanted.

Metabolic Transformation also works within my schedule and is not overly rigid. It provides the flexibility of my personal macronutritional range and utilizes what I want to eat, within reason. (My wife states that when they come out with the "all-carb diet" to let her know.) I realized that I could get up early and exercise and that I didn't have to lift weights three or four days a week (two days are fine) to get stronger and help burn fat. It's also just as satisfying to order the salmon and veggies with no butter than a cheeseburger and fries once you have created the discipline of healthy habits. Actually, it's more satisfying because you walk away with a mental victory and physical progress toward your goal. In the past, I was in the rut of ordering the double cheeseburger, large fries, and large soda when I went out for lunch. Always the same thing; never deviated. Now it's a small sub (heavy on the veggies), baked chips (if any), and water. Discipline is not a bad word. Discipline in the area of eating will develop joy and confidence that carries over to other aspects of your life. You will see that you can indeed conquer those seemingly insurmountable pounds.

I find that by eating three times a day and having two snacks that my blood sugar is much better balanced. I have great energy all day, and since this program is more moderate in carbs (unlike some other rigid anti-carb plans), I have the mental sharpness that I need. Carbohydrates are necessary to power the brain and nervous system whereas ketone bodies (the byproducts of an ultra-low carb diet) have a terrible time crossing the blood-brain barrier. That's why you feel like a walking zombie on low-carb diets—headachy and lethargic. I have no caffeine during the week, and I have gone from three Mountain Dews a day to one on Friday as a reward for making it through the week (this is America, isn't it?). Understand that even the most disciplined athlete needs rest. You will enjoy a "splurge meal" once a week so you don't feel like you have to deprive yourself 24/7.

In the past I was plagued with various ailments, which I always attributed to my constant exposure to illness in my practice. However, these past years I have been healthy and strong. I believe primarily this has been as a result of *Metabolic Transformation*. This book will help give you the information to prepare yourself to eat healthy the rest of your life. Most of us pay better attention to the type of oil and gas that go into our car than what we put in our mouths. It's time to change.

You have to decide. Joe often says there are two types of clients who come into his office: one who is determined to do anything it takes to achieve his or her goals, and one who is constantly looking to cut corners and see what he or she can get away with. If something is important to us, we will read every book, magazine, pamphlet, and Internet article we can find to help reach our goal. This book has the information; it has the goods, and no one will try to move your cheese. They also said on *Diet Wars*, "No one ever got rich by marketing self-control." However, self-control is where it starts. I had a hard time committing to the program when I was lifting weights and there were women half my size lifting more than I was. Then I realized that it wasn't about ego. It's not about the bully kicking sand in your face at the beach (my apologies, Mr. Atlas), and it sure as heck isn't about the next high-school reunion reality show. This is real life. It's about health. There is no amount of money that can replace your health. You picked up this book, didn't you? I believe that your life is worth at least $25, don't you? (Maybe if you're Canadian your life is worth $29.99.) It is impossible to be completely inclusive in any single piece of media, but we have tried to create something that will serve as a reference to come back to throughout life. It is not merely a 10-page pamphlet expanded, but a compilation of years of clinical experience and the assimilation of nutritional research. Attainable and sustainable.

You spent your hard-earned money for the book, and I sincerely hope you take the time and energy to follow the program and put it into practice. After a few weeks of results, you'll realize it was worth it. Make up your mind. No one else will do it for you. You are not dead yet. Don't be a casualty of doing nothing. Joe and I are here to support you, and you will succeed. And not just for today, but for a lifetime. Don't be intimidated. Get busy living!

CHAPTER ONE

GETTING STARTED

"Okay, Maggot! Get in here! Prepare to eat tofu, tree bark, and birdseed and like it! Prepare for pain and lots of it, Mr. Chicken-Wings-for-Arms. Now drop and give me 20 or until you puke, which ever comes last, you soda-guzzling, cheese curl-munching pud!" I guess that's kind of what I expected the first time I walked into Club Fitness Zone, the first serious gym I had attended since college. I expected to find a conglomeration of jock stereotypes just waiting to give me a wedgie, or worse, having to get me dislodged from some piece of equipment that I had no idea how to use. ("Hey, the new guy got himself caught in the Hamstring Strangulator again. What a weenie. It's your turn to get him out.")

What I found, however, was a group of people much like myself who were more concerned with camaraderie and their own health than watching someone else screw up. The local sheriff, attorneys, teachers, businessmen, and work-at-home moms were all there trying to improve their health. Many of them had similar stories of how they had overcome their own weight-loss demons. One gentleman had lowered his triglycerides from 900 to 90. A middle-aged woman had lost 60 pounds and kept it off. Another person had rehabbed from debilitating back problems. Each person had a different story, but each was clear about the goals he or she wanted to achieve. The main point I am trying to emphasize is *don't be intimidated*. Whether you decide to work out at the local gym or exercise at home where your wife and kids may make fun of your Spandex, others have been there and want you to succeed. The important thing is just getting started. You will make mistakes, but you need to learn to forgive yourself. Fitness is a marathon, not a sprint.

On this diet you will eat healthy, normal food that you can find at any grocery store. (Don't you hate when diet books or infomercials say that? Like we are going to spend time eating a lot of abnormal food that we had shipped over from Chernobyl.) Let me emphasize "healthy." I am not promising you that you can feast on steaks and lobster tails unless they are in small, normal portions. If you don't already eat in a healthy manner then be prepared to spend a little extra time on your initial runs to the store in order to begin to formulate some new shopping patterns. It will take longer to examine food labels and to prepare fruits and veggies, but just like anything else that's worthwhile, the time you invest will reap huge rewards down the road.

The Basics

To begin, you have to know what the macronutrients are. They are protein, carbohydrates (or carbs), and fat. Now, that was a difficult lesson, wasn't it? I could try to impress you with a detailed explanation of all of this, but we'll save that for later on.

The macronutrients are counted in grams per serving and are listed right on the side of any package, except most alcohol. If you don't learn to read labels you will be fooled constantly. Create the habit of flipping to the label and scanning the nutrients as well as the portion size. Knowing the value of what you put in your body is crucially important so do not overlook this critical step.

Be Prepared Mentally

You must change the way you think about food. As Joe likes to remind me, "A little hunger won't kill you." However, Americans have become conditioned that we shouldn't be hungry for a millisecond or have to lift a finger to achieve fitness. The models on the infomercials may have prepared with discipline and hours of hard work, or they may have achieved that look by unhealthy habits or multiple visits to the local plastic surgeon. Your anatomy is your anatomy and your goals are your goals. I will never, ever have arms like Joe's even if I lift weights until I'm 80. However, he will never be as tall as I am. Ha! Okay, I'd rather trade my height for his arms; however, the fact that I am not blessed with a certain physique does not stop me from going to the gym and trying my best. This is about health and self-improvement. As soon as you learn to accept your genes, you'll be much happier trying to maximize your potential. Don't waste your life agonizing over your supposed flaws. Even the most "beautiful people" constantly want someone else's lips, buns, or chest. You are "fearfully and wonderfully made," so work on the best *you* that you can be. It is called *Metabolic Transformation* not *Celebrity Transformation*. The good news is that this book will give you the shortcuts and information you need so that you can achieve weight loss as well as a higher level of fitness. But just like the proverbial swampland in Florida, beware of any other programs that sound too good to be true. Any program that tells you that you won't have to diet or exercise to achieve your goals is a complete lie. Have you ever really known anyone that successfully "burned calories while they slept?" Give me a break. Those programs are deceptive and only lead to despair among the chronic dieters who try them. *Metabolic Transformation* is based on scientific facts and can help you turn your life around if you are dedicated to changing your bad habits. You are not a failure, but you do have to toughen up a little. You are stronger than you think you are!

As you decrease your carbs and until you create the habits to get adequate protein in your diet, you will have a few days of feeling run down. However, there is not an overwhelming number of those days. Typically they pass in less that a week. *Transformation* is more about moderation. You will not be asked to go like a sports car into a brick wall by cutting your usual 300 carbs a day to 25 overnight. Ask any of your Atkinsian friends (is that like Dickensian? "Please sir, can I have some more butter on my steak?") how well their brain functioned on 25 carbs a day or how long they were able to sustain it. When you follow our plan (The Diet Docs' Rx), and consume a more reasonable amount of carbs with protein, you will have a good level of energy and your hunger will be very manageable. If you ever experience a tiny hunger pang at the end of the night it may signal that you will have a good morning on the scale rather than going to bed overly full and watching those little red numbers go up. Furthermore, hunger will truly fade as your body transitions to faster levels of body fat loss.

For my soda-guzzling friends: you folks will have to get off the sauce. Many of us would site the inevitable "caffeine headache" as to why we couldn't or wouldn't stop our intake. There are 40 to 45 carbs in a 12-ounce can and a mind-numbing 75 grams in a 20-ounce bottle, which is 30 to 50% of what your daily carb intake should be. A 44-ounce convenience store fountain drink has enough sugar to power a small country! If you are truly serious about losing weight, you must kick the soda habit. You really won't be able to afford even one can a day on this program. That huge sugar load will send your insulin levels through the roof and will lead to fat storage. One study shows that merely 1 can a day of regular pop can cause you to gain 15 pounds over the course of a year! Even more serious is the impact on your pancreas and insulin receptor sites. The constant sugar loading may seem like a harmless habit, but you're laying the groundwork for diabetes. I'm warning you: don't "Do the Dew."

I found that when I ate enough protein during the day, I never had a "caffeine headache." I don't like coffee or tea so I never substituted that. I believe some of the headaches people experience are actually hypoglycemia, and when their blood sugar is better balanced, they do not have as severe a problem with "withdrawal headaches." I once asked my friends who had been engineers at a soda manufacturer if they put something addictive in their product, and they said, "Yeah, sugar and caffeine." "No way, my learned-friends," I said, "there must be some kind of secret addictive ingredient, a chemical X, that keeps you hooked." "Yeah," they said, "sugar and caffeine." Work on getting rid of soda and other sugary drinks. Water is the healthiest drink you can put in your body. There is indeed a reason that your body and this planet are made up of so much of it—it's good for you!

See Your Physician

Now this is not just put in here to give the lawyers something to do; this is a critical part of your total health. It's hard to tell if you have high blood pressure or thyroid problems or anything else for that matter if you don't get checked. You can get cholesterol screenings and blood pressure checks at work, health fairs, or church, but that is no substitute for a thorough review by a physician. Most of us simply don't want to go to our physicians because we don't want them to lecture us like parents about our poor health habits. ("Now Johnny, you need to quit smoking two packs a day and eating all those two-pound triple cheeseburgers. Your mother and I have decided no dessert or Cartoon Network for a week if you can't cut back.") I know I didn't see my physician for a couple of years because I didn't want to hear it either. We all prefer to camp out by that river in Egypt, De Nile. It is nestled right next to the crumbling ruins of the food pyramids. However, at some point in time, we all have to grow up and take responsibility for our own nutritional choices. The statute of limitations on parental dietary misconduct has expired. Some of us ate or didn't eat to spite our parents, and several people have succeeded despite terrible parental examples, so let's give our parents a break. Give yourself a break. Now this doesn't cover problems that stem from major depression, eating disorders, or other serious mental health issues. That is beyond the scope of this book and requires long-term follow up with your physician and/or counselor. If you suffer from one of these debilitating illnesses, I strongly encourage you to find someone you are comfortable with and work with them. Serious problems like those will take time to resolve. Do not give up. We want you to succeed.

Your doctor is your partner and not your parent. You need to be monitored and have someone in your corner to help encourage you long-term. If you discover that you have a problem, you and your doctor can work together to defeat it rather than being pulled under the water of De Nile by one of those currents of hypertension, diabetes, or coronary artery disease. To those of you who have already discussed your weight issues with your doctor and wouldn't miss a yearly physical, great job! Keep it up and ignore my previous ranting. A wise person seeks out correction, and I hope that we all try to be wise. Furthermore, do *not* ask for diet drugs to "jump start" your weight loss. You do not need them. You will likely lose five to seven pounds in the first week so you don't need a prescription. These medications are not without side effects (check with the Phen/Fen people) and you can only take them for a certain period of time under law. Time and again I see people take diet drugs, lose a few pounds, and one year later they are back to their previous weight and asking for the same darn thing. Even gastric bypass, which can be a life-changing operation, does have its risks. I have seen people lose 100 pounds or more on this program without resorting to something as dramatic as surgery. If you apply the principles in these pages, you will lose five to seven pounds in the first week and one to two pounds a week thereafter. It may not be a quick fix, but it is the healthy, sensible way to lose weight. Better yet, it will help you learn to change your habits and it won't harm your metabolism, which will make it easier to keep the weight off for good.

If you need a friend or a loved one to give you a hand, ask them. However, and this is very important, it is *your* responsibility to lose weight and no one else's. If you are really serious, you don't need to tell your friends, neighbors, or your cat that you are going on a diet. You don't really need to have anyone other than yourself to hold you accountable. The only one you would cheat is yourself. Let's face it, "Food eaten in secret tastes delicious." (Proverbs 9:17) They understood that 3,000 years ago and the Thighmaster hadn't even been invented yet. Let's say it again: the only one who holds you accountable is you. Not your parent, your spouse, your friends, or coworkers. You can nibble that cheesecake when your accountability partner isn't there, but the calories still count. You haven't fooled anyone when you step on the scale and wonder why "this diet just isn't working." Hmm, wonder why. The only exception to this rule is if your accountability partner were the latest TV fitness personality, and he or she would come over to your house and strap you into their latest piece of exercise equipment, the Ab/Bun/Thigh/Jackknife-o-Nator 3000, and scream at you for an hour. That would be motivation for anyone.

Preparing for Battle

Now a list of some things that will be helpful as you get started. This is, of course, not the only list. As you move along the program, we would love to hear what things you use to keep rolling along.

First, read this book all the way through. It seems like that should be fairly obvious, but I have known plenty of people who have abandoned a diet book because it was too complicated or just too darn boring. Hopefully, this book is neither and can be read in a weekend. Only a complete understanding of the principles in this book will allow you to apply these strategies repeatedly and effectively. We need to overcome not just "junk food" of the body but "junk food" of the mind as well. It's easy to click the remote endlessly at night or flip through the magazines in the check-out aisle, mentally digesting bits and pieces that dull our minds and sap our desire. You need to focus on this book and work to bring yourself to a good place mentally. Develop the discipline. Begin by reading this book cover to cover.

Second, start to gather your basic provisions, and trust me that this journey won't be as difficult as the Donner party. Here are some things I have found helpful:

1. A digital food scale of decent quality. Some people would say that having a scale is a little obsessive, but can you accurately tell what four ounces of meat is or what one ounce of nuts is? People will use the "size of a fist" or the "size of a deck of cards" thing, and that is helpful in a pinch, but I guarantee I can make my fist smaller or much, much larger depending on how hungry I am. If you are going to develop healthy eating habits, I believe it is critical to weigh your food when you can, especially in the early phases of your diet. I have discovered after weighing my meals that I often underestimated the amount of food I had by anywhere from 50 to 150%! Take the guesswork out of the picture. Be precise. Estimating rather than weighing may not make a lot of difference if you are eating tuna, but it could mean the difference of 10 versus 20 grams of fat if you are eating some red meat. Serving size has been so distorted by restaurant entrées that weighing is a good way to get things back in perspective and achieve a true portion size. Don't want to take a scale to work? Then don't. Weigh food in the morning or evening or on the weekends (just not in the shower or on the dashboard on the way to work). After awhile you will have a much easier time estimating true portion sizes of the foods you eat regularly.

2. Purchase proper measuring cups to help with your estimation. (For the culinary impaired, know there is a difference between measuring cups for solids and liquids.) I was very naïve about cooking (Hamburger Helper, Dinty Moore Beef Stew, and spaghetti were about all I could manage in college), and didn't realize that one fluid ounce does not equal one ounce by weight no matter how many times my eighth-grade Home Economics teacher told me the difference. Hey, the Food Network hadn't been invented when I was in college (which is a darn good thing or I would have missed a lot of classes sitting around watching Rachel Ray). One cup of a dry cereal by volume does not equal eight ounces by weight. There

are usually only 14 ounces in a box. This may seem elementary, but I once had a college roommate who used to eat his cereal out of a mixing bowl. He, of course, went on to achieve a Ph.D. in physics. My former breakfast routine seemed healthy, but upon closer examination, was just the opposite. I would pour my orange juice in a travel mug and run out the door to work. I thought I had about 8 ounces, but when I actually measured, it was 12 ounces. Then when I read the label and found out how much sugar is in juice, combined with the high number of carbs in my breakfast bar, it wasn't hard to figure out part of why my weight loss was slowed. That little science experiment only took a few minutes to calculate, but it taught me a very valuable lesson.

3. Get a journal. Doesn't matter what kind. You just have to be faithful to write down whatever goes in your mouth. It is a truism in medicine—document everything. This is not obsessive—it is a semi-objective way to see where you might be having problems. Develop the discipline of writing it down. Those little candy bar miniatures add up when you eat several a day. The difference in 200 carbs versus 125 is very substantial over time. Also, a journal is useful for keeping track of your exercise and any random notes of encouragement to yourself. You don't have to buy anything expensive. I usually obtain a devotional journal that has blank pages and jot down columns for protein, carbs, and fat and add them up as the day goes on.

4. Although I joked about it earlier, unless you are good at adding things in your head, get an inexpensive calculator to add your totals of your three macronutrients. Keep it simple.

5. Get a food counter book. These usually are sold in the diet section of your local bookstore and cost about $8. It will help you estimate or even give you the true nutritional values for many items. If you are not sure about the value of a certain item and you know it may have a lot of fat or carbs, be careful. Take a small portion of it. Don't sabotage yourself.

6. To weigh or not to weigh, that is the question. Whether 'tis nobler to watch thy downward progress or to wail at the upward slide of the needle—I don't have a good answer to that one, folks. I have already talked about my love/hate relationship with my scale, but haven't thrown it out the window yet. For me, a scale was a good tool to learn what foods affected me and what I could do to combat the upward slide. For example, I learned that I was more sensitive to fat calories than carbs and if I over did it on my fat intake, I would gain weight and it would take much longer to lose than if I overate a little on my carbs. I liked to weigh daily initially because it helped inspire me and it helped establish new healthy habits (walk, weigh, hit the showers, then prepare for a day of healthy eating). If you are going to weigh,

then use the same scale at the same time of the day with the same amount of clothing. Most people find that a salty meal will show up on the scale the next morning. Women will find their weight increasing due to water retention during their monthly cycle. Whatever you do with regard to using the scale, keep going. Don't be discouraged. If you are consistent, the weight will come off. Be objective. Don't wander from scale to scale until you find one that makes you feel a little better. You are tracking trends, so be consistent and use the same instrument. Some people, however, allow their scale to control their mood, which goes up and down based on those little red numbers. If you can't handle the truth and a "bad scale day" will send you into the "I-suck-so-I'll-just-eat-an-entire-pan-of-brownies" state of mind, then don't weigh daily or don't even weigh at all. To thine own self be true. Know yourself and your limitations so that the scale is a tool simply like a book or a measuring cup, and do not let it control you. It's not a mechanical judge of your self worth.

Wow, what a complicated list! Run to your local store, get stocked, and get ready. Some will think to skip this step. "I'm smarter than the average reader; I'll just read the book and implement some of the ideas." Come on. Your wife may program the DVD player for you and rebuild the kids' toys when you don't read the directions, but this is important. Don't skip things; play by the rules.

Read the Labels

This sounds totally obvious doesn't it? (So obvious that I mention it twice in this chapter.) However, get into the habit of doing it routinely. That "Nutrition Facts" panel on the side of the box is your friend. The government mandates it to be on every package, so take advantage of that. (How often do you get anything free, other than cheese, from the government?) Pay particular attention to serving size. Is it five nuggets or six? It may not seem like much, but that's a 20% difference. Even what you think would be an obvious serving size may actually be two servings or even two and a half. Drinks, especially soda, are notorious for that. The 20-ounce bottle is 2.5 8-ounce servings so that if you drink it all, you have to multiply the carbs and calories by 2.5. Seems just a little sneaky, doesn't it? I once ate a certain flatbread sandwich for a whole week and patted myself on the back for being so good. I kept thinking that it tasted too good and filling to be so low in carbs. I finally looked at the label only to discover that each wrap was actually two servings! That reminds me of a diet strategy that one of my patients told me. His aged family doctor told him there was an easy method to lose weight: if you put something in your mouth and it tastes good, spit it out.

It's obviously not good for you. Lucky for us, with modern food science and creative recipe books, that doesn't always have to be true. You can handle the truth—don't ignore the label.

Exercise

Now this is a fun part! Whether you like to or not, you need to exercise. Let me stress the importance of fitness. A successful weight-loss plan must include some form of repeated physical activity. Many people find that when they start exercising regularly that they actually (gasp!) like it. The multiple health benefits of exercise do not need to be debated here. From a clinical perspective I can tell you that my most fit elderly patients have "taken some exercise" for decades, and I have some 70-and 80-year-olds that can do push ups like Jack Palance on Oscar night. Put some thought into this exercise thing. I cringe when I think about the hundreds of dollars wasted on equipment and gym memberships that I never used. Even though it may seem like a good deal; never get a lifetime membership to a gym unless they are extremely well-established. (I've had two gyms close after I had signed up for "lifetime" memberships. It was starting to give me a complex.) Do whatever works, but don't buy a thousand-dollar treadmill and let it sit idle as a clothes rack in your basement. Joe and I are strong believers that you need both cardiovascular training—such as walking, running, or bike riding—in addition to some type of strength training to accelerate your weight loss. A few other people in the United States probably believe that too and here's why. If your muscles are fit, you will be burning more calories even at rest. Read that last sentence again. You can lose weight with diet alone, cardio alone, lifting alone, or a combination of all three. However, if you want to have the greatest level of total fitness and not look just like a deflated balloon from dieting alone, you need all three. I still suffer from "deflated balloon belly," but hey, I'm working on it! Of course ol' "Washboard Joe" wouldn't know what I was talking about. Skinny overachiever. Scour the paper for an inexpensive set of weights, use a reputable video program, or join a gym. Hey, we give you flexibility with your food *and* your workouts!

Gyms often will have introductory deals where you can work with a trainer for several sessions. Look for one who is certified and dig into their experience level. The National Strength and Conditioning Association (NSCA) has stringent certification guidelines. (Maybe if you are a little timid an ASPCA trainer would be more up your alley.) Remember that *you* are the consumer. Some trainers want to impress you by how sore they can make you the next day. "Well if I can't walk, I must have really gotten a good workout." The only thing that type of "training" leads to is injury and burn-out. Take your time and let them know if it is too much weight to lift. By and large trainers are fine people who want to see you succeed because that makes you look good, them look good, and their gym owners look good. Friends can help, but it is better to work with a trainer or physical therapist who understands different ways to do an exercise to prevent injury or take stress off a particular joint. Get an inexpensive start after you consult your physician of course (we can't have all those lawyers sitting around with nothing to do, can we? Someone might get a spare lawsuit in the eye).

True, you can lose weight without exercise (good nutrition takes care of that), and to someone who is gravely obese or disabled, this book is very important. However, for the majority of us who are able to exercise, it is crucial that we move. It is about achieving total health for the skeleton, cardiovascular system, lungs, and entire body. It is also very possible to exercise regularly and not have a good nutritional plan and be an "in-shape fat person." Many of us know someone who never missed a session at the gym but is still carrying 40 to 50 pounds too much. Often I would see that same person hit the vending machine before he left the gym. These people labor under the misconception that the 30 to 60 minutes of exercise will offset a day's worth of poor nutritional choices. Granted, they are better off than if they were doing nothing. But let's face it: if you are going to work that hard, you want to achieve complete total health and not complete self-deception. Being stronger, more athletic, and looking better is just an added bonus. If you "don't have time" to exercise you are shortening your life span and decreasing your overall quality of life. Ultimately your time will be up sooner than you think.

Knowing Your Enemy and Arming Yourself

This is the bulk of what this book is about. I frankly view this as answering Dr. Agatston's challenge. You know; the guy who wrote *The South Beach Diet*. He has issued the somewhat snickering challenge "unless someone popularizes the science of nutrition" we have to rely a bit on the diet du jour. Well, guess what, doc? We are here to do just that. Nutrition should be popular and we're here to make the science understandable and accessible. That should be your goal. Understanding nutrition is the only way to adjust your eating habits no matter what challenges are facing you on the job, at home, or on the go.

We have already discussed reading the labels. You should do that with every food product in your kitchen. (Are Twinkies considered a food product?) Write the nutritional numbers down. Also, as you prepare food, keep the packages and calculate the values of a serving size of a casserole or similar product. This will take a little bit of work, but it is well worth it. I discovered I could eat my wife's homemade tomato and basil pizza, but I could only have two pieces instead of my usual three or four. Try to plan ahead for nights when you might eat more fat or carbs. Be flexible with your meal preparation. It really helped to watch my fat and carb intake during the day so I could afford that wonderful pizza occasionally. It drives me crazy when I see a diet book that talks about virtually unlimited pizza and beer like you are back in college. Although those types of foods may be one of the great sensual pleasures of life, too much of them has added to the obesity problem in the first place! And if you are eating in an unhealthy manner and simply "exercising the calories away," you are still not doing your body or your immune system any favors.

We are not going to make any inane promises about how you can just eat anything anytime and still lose weight. We eat a lot of healthy food and a small amount of not-so-healthy food to lose unwanted fat and achieve our goal weight. But, the key is having the right plan and sticking to it. You have to have your house stocked with plenty of nutritious snacks/meals that you can grab quickly when you are enticed to slam down the latest high-fat, high-carb temptation. A common excuse is that "there was nothing else in the house/office/machine/car or my kid's lunchbox." Plan ahead and prepare for success. Keep protein bars, shakes, mixed nuts, tuna, hard-boiled eggs, and whole-grain/whole-food carb sources on hand to help defeat the cravings. As you gain some experience, you'll discover what foods you have a hard time getting into your diet, and which foods trigger cravings. You'll have to plan better to have some foods available, and you may find you need to avoid some like the plague. I made a game out of trying new foods that I had never eaten before and watching people's expressions as I ate them ("Ostrich jerky? Eww!"). People who say they don't have the time must get serious and learn to make time. All of us have time for things that are important. A little planning (such as buying things in bulk or cooking ahead) may save you on a day when you are really in a hurry, which today is just about every day. Make your shopping trips more like *The Purpose Driven Life* than *A Series of Unfortunate Events*.

Stick with It/Be Patient

You may have a white-collar job, but in order to succeed you have to have a blue-collar work ethic. Don't cheat yourself out of your share of life! Though a cliché, you didn't gain it overnight so you shouldn't expect to lose it overnight. Every legitimate publication says that safe weight loss is one to two pounds per week, max. If you have 50 to 60 pounds to lose you must accept it will take 6 or more months to lose the weight safely. Don't give up after 90 days. Keep on keeping on. You may hit plateaus and it may take several weeks to break through them. In the process of my weight loss, I hit two plateaus. One took three weeks to defeat and the other took four. Stick with it and you will smash through.

"Experts" may disagree on the methods to lose weight, but there are some things on which everyone can agree: you must cut calories, decrease fat intake, and restrict carbs. *Metabolic Transformation* does these three things while stressing whole grains, fruits, and vegetables in an amount that won't leave your glucose-hungry brain deprived. Combined with all the other tools we give you, *your* results can be consistent, permanent, and at the same time, flexible.

Eat!

Sounds kind of contradictory for a diet book, doesn't it? You will have to eat, and at times you will seem like you are eating more than you did when you were "dieting" in the past. You must eat enough in your optimal range to activate your metabolic transformation.

You need to *stay ahead of hunger*. You will need to eat your meals and your snacks even if you don't feel hungry. If you put too much time between meals or snacks, your blood sugar will drop and you will feel hungry, therefore tempted to binge. Don't do that—plan ahead. Create new healthy habits to replace your bad habits. Much of eating is habitual, and you will be shocked how easy it is to replace that pink coconut marshmallow ball thing with a protein bar. You've seen the consequences of impulsive and unwise choices. However, junk food will always be out there. It's not like you'll never get to eat any for the rest of your life. Remember that old Doritos commercial with Jay Leno? The tag line was something like, "Eat all you want; we'll make more." Well of course they will! It's not like the supply of junk food will ever go away in this country. It's a matter of deciding that you will no longer continue to eat junk if you want to be healthy. Send a message to the junk food industry. There are alternatives to sugar and trans-fats and we want them! It will take you only a matter of weeks to change if you focus. Do your own shopping. Again, don't rely on anyone else to take care of your responsibilities. Remember that you are trying to become your own nutritionist. Read the labels. Know where the healthy food can be found in the store and which stores carry the freshest ingredients. Avoid processed foods such as crackers, chips, and cookies. Sure they taste good, but once you open a bag it is difficult to put it down. These processed foods cause huge releases of insulin, which will drive your body to place excess calories into fat cells and put your pancreas under unbelievable strain. That important organ, buried deep in the middle of your abdomen, will finally say "No mas" and will stop functioning properly. When that happens, you will get type II (adult onset) diabetes. It is that simple. I frequently tell people in my practice that it is like running your car too close to the red line for too long a period of time; eventually things will break and parts will start falling off. I believe that people think that with our current medical technology that we can "cure" diabetes—or any other illness for that matter. We do have medicines to treat the disease better, but because of our increasing weight, diabetes is growing at epidemic proportions, and it is still a leading cause of blindness, kidney failure, heart attacks, and amputations. Are the three sodas a day worth the loss of your leg? Put good fuel in your tank and meals will be a pleasure and an adventure instead of another opportunity for failure and advancement of certain diseases.

I used to roll my eyes when people would tell me they "didn't eat anything" but couldn't lose weight. One of the reasons was simply that they didn't eat enough. They basically tricked their bodies into thinking they were starving, and their bodies tried as hard as they could to hold on to the few calories they were taking in. These people may need to eat more to lose weight.

Many, though, think they're not eating much, but because they're not tracking it, they have no idea that their food intake is actually high enough to impair fat loss. The purpose of *Metabolic Transformation* is to show you how to eat the proper amounts to accelerate your weight loss instead of stalling it out or failing at it due to lack of knowledge. This is where The Diet Docs' Rx comes in. Curious about what this Rx thing is that we've been talking about? Well come with me, my friend. Get ready to get transformed, and put down that bag of cheese puffs!

CHAPTER ONE KEY POINTS

▸ 1) Metabolic Transformation is based on solid science.

▸ 2) Be can active participant in your success.

▸ 3) No one is the same metabolically or personally. While providing the right structure, Metabolic Transformation allows maximum flexibility.

▸ 4) See your physician for a physical – you're overdue.

▸ 5) Take responsibility, be consistent, track your food, learn, and permanent success will be yours.

CHAPTER TWO

THE DIET DOCS' RX

Metabolism Defined

Not long ago, a 44-year-old man came to me with a goal of getting leaner and possibly gaining some muscle. He already enjoyed a lifestyle of working out and running almost every day and had done so for most of his adult life. Despite being very healthy from his physical training perspective, he gained and lost 20 pounds more than once and lamented his lack of control. He wanted to lose weight again, but he also wanted a permanent change and permanent control. This, of course, forces thoughts of success as a mental obstacle. Perhaps my client needed a master motivator to drive his consciousness into a higher level of passion regarding his abs and biceps. Perhaps I could hypnotize him and plant subconscious links between snack cakes and rat poison. Instead, I've found the greatest link to success is to help people get their metabolic physiology in order, and in the process teach them how and why they are doing it. There is an intertwining of the physiological and the psychological aspects of weight loss that cannot be separated. A great number of failed dieters feel tremendous guilt about not being disciplined when it may be simply that they don't understand the physiology of what's happening and what they can do to positively affect it. I can't tell you how many times I've heard, "I have control over every aspect of my life except my weight. Why?!" The physical and mental sides of diet affect each other in a very dynamic relationship. As you'll learn in the rest of this chapter, the first week of changing your nutrition brings about significant changes in your body internally, literally creating stability that makes it easier than you think to not only lose weight, but to do it without suffering. *Attainable and sustainable* is the phrase you can use to describe *Metabolic Transformation*.

My new client lost 20 pounds of body fat and gained 5 pounds of lean muscle mass in his first 8 weeks. How can a man who already exercises regularly, works out with weights at least four days per week, and runs in road races have such dramatic results just by changing his nutrition? The answer is metabolism. He actually complained of having to eat so much food on his program, yet after these first eight weeks I had to increase his food so he wouldn't lose weight "too quickly." He often commented on his new, higher level of energy. A very disciplined, in-control person, he went as far as saying, "Coming to you literally changed my life." Are these the typical comments of dieters you know? Study after study has shown most dieters regain even more weight than they lose on any given plan. We are here to break that mold! We're going to set you up for permanent results, not just a temporary fix.

How many times have you heard people say they have a fast or slow metabolism? Thin people often say, "I have a fast metabolism," and those who are overweight often say, "I have a slow metabolism." We are quick to blame or credit our body size on a word that most of us don't understand. Basal metabolic rate is the rate at which your body burns calories over a specific amount of time. It's true that there is some variability in everyone's metabolism; however, I have met few people who had a legitimately "slow" metabolism due to a thyroid imbalance, metabolic condition, or medical ailment that would compromise weight loss. In other words, your metabolism may be slightly lower than someone else's, but it is probably not the reason you are overweight.

The cause of your weight struggle likely goes beyond your genetic metabolism; though for a small percentage of people, genetics do play a major role in making it easier to gain weight. Hormone levels that were immeasurable just years ago are being found to be major players in weight loss and gain. These hormones directly control metabolism, fat storage, and even hunger levels. The number of genetic fat cells can even be significantly different between people making it harder for some to lose weight. There is great research being done on morbid obesity that will help a lot of people, but most of us are overweight by our own eating habits.

Don't misunderstand me. While I'm downplaying the role of metabolism as an excuse, it does play a great role with long-term impact in the big picture of weight management. What you eat *does* affect your metabolism. Within weeks, you can raise or lower your body's ability to burn calories, sometimes significantly. Over time, this change can add up to large weight loss or gain. To be quite honest, this is the foundation of permanent weight loss. By eating the right amount of food, eating within the right daily structure, consuming better ratios of the three macronutrients (protein, carbohydrates, and fat), selecting the right food choices, and learning to be consistent, you can actually increase the amount of calories your body burns per day. This change in metabolism is due to the optimum operation of your body's internal environment.

(Figure 2:1) Basal Metabolic Rate

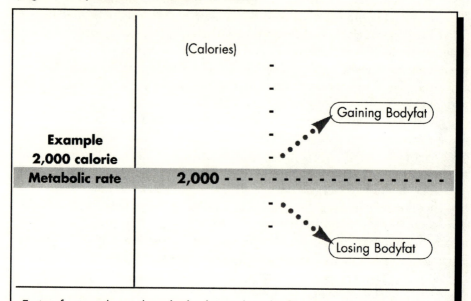

Eating fewer calories than the body needs is the first step to losing weight, however, done improperly will cause the body to decrease calorie burning making it easier to gain body fat. Permanent, positive changes in metabolism will occur only through the combined results of eating nutrients in the right amounts in a structured meal plan.

When you diet or eat incorrectly, your body does not work at optimum levels. Know anyone who has lost 30 pounds only to gain 40 back? They may insist they didn't gorge themselves to regain the weight but simply started eating "normally." Incorrect dieting can reduce the amount of calories your body burns, therefore making it much easier to gain weight even though you're trying to lose weight. Pay close attention to the details of this book as we explore how your body works with correct eating and diet.

AVERAGE JOE PHYSIOLOGY

The Straight Scoop on Metabolism

Numerous studies show how quickly our bodies can be affe___ changes in diet. The dreaded "slow metabolism" isn't to be blamed ___ of us; the super-sized lunches, chips, snacks, double helpings at dinne___ ___nd the worn track from the couch to the kitchen are the real culprits. But when we chose to embark on a weight-loss plan, we can do some short-term damage to our metabolism by incorrect eating.

A study showed that after 24 days of low-calorie dieting (450 calories – that's low!) the metabolism can be decreased by 15%. Several studies have reported decreases in resting metabolic rate up to 20 to 30%. Dropping your metabolism that fast means you're likely to regain more weight back when you start "eating normally" again until your metabolism catches back up, which it will do. In extreme cases, such as anorexia, metabolic rates have been measured to be slashed by 45%.

You may not be aware that just as eating too little decreases your metabolic rate, overeating increases it. This is where we lose the "I'm fat because of a slow metabolism" excuse. One study showed that when subjects who required 3,100 calories to maintain their weight gained 20% or more of their initial weight, they had to eat 5,100 calories to maintain that extra weight due to a heightened metabolism. (That gives credence to some who say, "I don't eat enough, that's why I can't lose weight." The metabolism is very sensitive and needs to sometimes be "rebuilt," but changes have to be made incrementally.

The importance of small changes is shown clearly in "yo-yo" dieting. Going on and off of diets repeatedly makes it more difficult to lose weight. Remember, the negative effects are short-term and your metabolism can be corrected, but the damage (weight regain) can be done so fast that you actually regain more weight than you lost. One study took subjects through two cycles of weight loss and weight regain. The rate of loss was only half during the second cycle compared to the first and the rate of regain was increased by 300%! That means when you diet and then binge and then diet again, you are only 50% as effective metabolically than the first round, and when your metabolism is suppressed from the dieting, you regain weight back 3 times faster than if you hadn't dieted at all. (That's how sensitive your metabolism is and why you need to have a knowledge base to guide you to successful and permanent weight loss. Scott got to experience this

continued ⟶

AVERAGE JOE PHYSIOLOGY

firsthand over the holidays when we first worked together. Already doing great with his weight loss, he thought, "Hey, I'm exercising, I'm doing great; I can eat all this sugar and fat and just burn it off." One dessert led to another, party after party, and 17 pounds later, reality set in. It took months to re-lose that weight and he learned that you can't outsmart your metabolism.

Eating the Right Amount to Raise Your Metabolism

As we progress through specific nutrient information and physiology, you will clearly see how the amount, type, and consumption pattern of food can literally accelerate your metabolism to full throttle. The first and most important step, however, is to estimate your metabolic rate correctly so you can eat the right amount of food that allows you to reach your weight-loss goals. Once you know how much energy your body requires, you can adjust your eating downward to begin the weight-loss process.

You could logically assume that eating 5 calories less than your body requires burns 5 extra calories stored as body fat, or that if you consume 500 calories less, your body makes up the difference by burning 500 calories of stored fat. Actually, the process is more complex than this. There is far more to permanent weight loss than just reducing calories. For instance, the body can burn calories by catabolizing, or breaking down, other tissues such as muscle. Even if your goals don't include gaining muscle, the last thing you want to do is lose lean body mass. Retaining muscle is too important for long-term metabolic function, strength, energy, and even in preventing osteoporosis. Other "intermediate" sources of energy such as blood sugar and stored carbohydrates (glycogen) in the liver and muscle may be used as well. Thus, the goal is to maximize fat loss while sparing muscle. There is a fine line between losing the most body fat as fast as possible and doing it in such a way that your metabolism is raised and not lowered.

The first step is to determine the right amount of food necessary to reach your goal. I have developed a chart based on gender and height to make this most important step very easy. This chart ensures enough food to avoid any deficiencies in the three macronutrients, and is geared towards a one-to-two pound weight loss per week.

(Figure 2:2) Metabolic Range

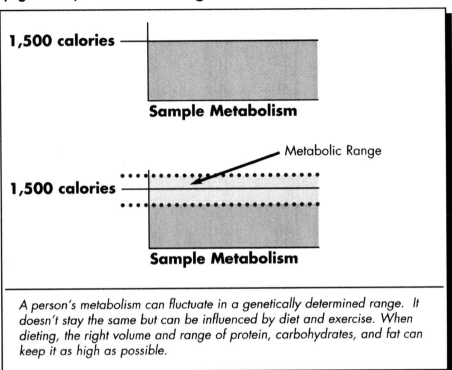

A person's metabolism can fluctuate in a genetically determined range. It doesn't stay the same but can be influenced by diet and exercise. When dieting, the right volume and range of protein, carbohydrates, and fat can keep it as high as possible.

A great deal of experience and human trial has been poured into this chart to make it simple as well as the most powerful tool you have ever had in your battle for permanent weight control. It seems too easy to just plug yourself into a chart and follow the numbers, but therein lies the challenge. It will require discipline to stay with your program. Most people reading this will not have a clear concept regarding the numbers on the chart. In other words, most cannot correlate how much food is required to eat 100 grams of protein or even what foods contain protein. Fear not: within six weeks you will be on the way to becoming your own nutritionist. Thousands of clients have found this plan to provide the most attainable and sustainable results ever experienced. A significant help is the flexibility you have in food selection yet the strict guidance you have in your personal macronutrient range profile. This chart is the cornerstone of the program. All of the science contained in the book is funneled into this tool, The Diet Docs' Rx.

So, there you have one of our most powerful tools and we didn't make you wait 20 chapters to find it. Those of you that want something simple; here it is. Eat within the levels appropriate for your gender and height and you'll lose weight. Thank you and good night. You and I both know, though, that it's more than just hitting a gram or calorie total. Knowing what to eat, how to structure your day nutritionally, plan meals, and learning about the individuality of your body is what pays dividends long after you set this book aside.

What if It Doesn't Seem to Be Working?

Everything we will explore from this point will define this one simple step of consuming the right amounts of the three macronutrients. We will expand and explain a great deal of information that will make this step even easier, yet it is still your responsibility to stay within the levels on this chart. It won't require weird foods (like pomegranate or grilled alligator) or crazy behaviors (like sit-ups hanging from your garage rafters or pushing a cart through snowy Russian mountains as in *Rocky IV*), just discipline. There are two very different definitions of the word discipline. The first is punishment. As soon as you read the word discipline related to weight loss, I know it sounds like punishment. However, the second definition is *your* definition: to train or develop by instruction; to impose order upon; orderly or prescribed conduct or pattern of behavior. That doesn't sound too hard does it? We want to train you in new habits that maximize your effort and health. It takes order and a pattern of behavior. We'll give you the prescription, and with the right motivation, we know you'll happily follow it with the promise of healthily attained permanent weight loss. Well, the last set of ab crunches may make you forget the "happily" part, but it will be worth it!

We have established that everyone is different metabolically, and therefore, this chart may not be a perfect fit for a few readers. The goal is to lose one to two pounds of body fat per week and this chart was created for the general population with a moderate activity level.

You may lose five to seven pounds the first week due to water loss, but one to two pounds each week thereafter is the goal. If, despite following your totals perfectly, eating the best food selections as described, and using the methods in this book, you are not obtaining the desired results, you may need to make an adjustment (Flexibility alert!). First, if you are not losing weight fast enough (one to two pounds per week) make sure you're eating at the low end of your macronutrient range. If you are losing too rapidly, make sure you're eating at the high end. If you're still losing too fast, add 25 grams of carbohydrates to your daily totals for a week and reassess your results. Keep adding until you are losing at the desired rate. If you are still losing too slowly even at the low end of your suggested chart totals, drop your daily intake of carbs by 10 grams daily for a week and reassess. If necessary, repeat this until you are losing weight at the appropriate rate.

(Figure 2:3) The Diet Docs' Rx (Personal Macronutrient Range)

Height	Men:	Women:
	(Grams per day)	
Under 5'		
Protein	100 - 120	60 - 80
Carbohydrates	120 - 150	80 - 110
Fat	35 - 40	20 - 25
(Calories)	(1,195 - 1,440)	(740 - 985)
5' - 5'4"		
Protein	110 - 130	70 - 90
Carbohydrates	130 - 160	90 - 120
Fat	40 - 45	25 - 30
(Calories)	(1,320 - 1,565)	(865 - 1,110)
5'5" - 5'8"		
Protein	120 - 140	80 - 100
Carbohydrates	140 - 170	100 - 130
Fat	45 - 50	30 - 35
(Calories)	(1,445 - 1,690)	(990 - 1,235)
5'9" - 6'		
Protein	130 - 150	90 - 110
Carbohydrates	150 - 180	110 - 140
Fat	50 - 55	35 - 40
(Calories)	(1,570 - 1,815)	(1,115 - 1,360)
6'1" - 6'4"		
Protein	140 - 160	100 - 120
Carbohydrates	160 - 190	120 - 150
Fat	55 - 60	40 - 45
(Calories)	(1,695 - 1,940)	(1,240 - 1,485)

What to Expect the First Week

As briefly mentioned, your body has many sources of energy to draw from. As anyone lowers calorie intake below what is necessary (basal metabolic rate), the caloric deficit must be made up from somewhere. Though we would all like it to be body fat that is used, there is actually a percentage of energy taken from almost every available source. The most readily available is blood sugar and then liver glycogen (stored sugar). These are dynamic, easy-to-access energy stores that are immediately used when needed.

(Figure 2:4) The First Step

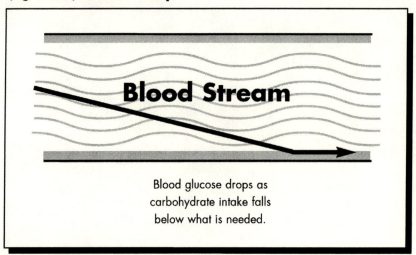

Blood glucose drops as carbohydrate intake falls below what is needed.

Muscle glycogen is a large area of stored energy but its primary purpose is for muscle contraction and work and is therefore not as easily retrieved for maintenance calorie needs.

Between meals, body fat is released from body fat cells, but only as much as is needed. So, if you follow the path, this paragraph will be monumental to your understanding. Your food intake is now precise and consistent so that you will get precise and consistent results. The total amount of calories is moderately lower than your body needs on a daily basis so that it requires a secondary source of calories. The first place your body is going to access is blood sugar, liver glycogen, and a moderate amount of available muscle glycogen (especially if you work out).

Metabolic Transformation in Action

> My life-changing experience with Dr. Joe Klemczewski has been a blessing of untold proportions! I have no doubt whatsoever that he was purposely placed in my life to bring me out of the spiraling downfall of my body's physical health as well as my lagging mental and emotional spirit.
>
> Growing up, throughout my twenties, and even into my mid-thirties, I had always been the envied one who could eat anything and never gain a pound. It was quite a blow to my ego when I started to see the pounds slowly (at first) starting to accumulate. I tried to rationalize that this was normal. After all, I was getting older, right? I went from weighing no more than 120 to around 140 pounds. You need a little extra weight as you get older, others would tell me.
>
> Then, health problems started to flare up – gallbladder removal, female/hormonal problems, back problems, etc. I was getting a bleak picture of the aging process – and the numbers on the scale continued to climb...
>
> The first time I heard of Joe was when my school district hired him to speak to the entire district staff about health and nutrition. Joe has a special ability and talent for taking his vast knowledge of the human body and nutrition and bringing it to a level of understanding that everyone can comprehend. I was extremely impressed and interested, but in my mind I was only slightly overweight at 160 pounds. Others assured me I was fine – but did I feel fine? The numbers on the scale continued to climb...
>
> The next time I heard about Joe was in my doctor's office, Dr. J. Scott Uloth, to whom, by the way, I am eternally grateful. At this point I need to express how Dr. Uloth has been a rock for me during some of the most difficult times of my life. On December 1, 2003, it was necessary for me to have a complete hysterectomy. On December 29 of that same month, my mother passed away unexpectedly, although she had recently been diagnosed with lung cancer. Ten months later, my mother-in-law died suddenly of a massive heart attack. Dr. Uloth listened, talked with me, and helped me through those difficult times. Words can never express my complete gratitude, Dr. Uloth. You are awesome! During this visit, I commented to Dr. Uloth about his own weight loss and overall look of good health. He began to talk to me enthusiastically about Dr. Joe and the help and encouragement he had been provided on his journey back to a healthy lifestyle. He gave me Joe's number and we continued my appointment for back and joint pain. At 174 pounds, the numbers on the scale continued to climb...
>
> continued ⟶

Metabolic Transformation in Action

March, 2004...Once again, I am at Dr. Uloth's office and I am once again running the gamut of aches, pains, illness, and emotions. I compliment Dr. Uloth on looking exceedingly healthy and trim. He, as usual, listened to me patiently, asked questions and looked over my chart. We dealt with my current complaint, of course, and then he broached the subject of my weight gain. My weight at that time was up to, I believe, 204 pounds. I had gained about 40 pounds from mid-December 2003 to March of 2004. We talked about the causes of the weight gain, both physical and emotional. At the age of 42, soon to be 43 years old, I had never felt so out of control in my life. I was trapped in an unhealthy body that didn't seem to respond to any of my many attempts to lose weight and improve my health. Dr. Uloth again mentioned all the positive effects of his work with Dr. Joe. I told him I was most definitely interested, but that it was an extremely busy time for me both at work and at home. I would be getting in touch with Dr. Joe after school was out in May. I left feeling more hopeful than I had in a while, but the numbers on the scale continued to climb...

On Wednesday, May 25, 2005, I had my first personal meeting with Dr. Joe. My weight had climbed to an unbelievable all-time high of 215 pounds! I was in an embarrassed, emotional state of mind and Dr. Joe had a very calming, reassuring manner. He talked with me for about two hours, explaining the importance of nutrition in weight loss, learning about my eating and exercise habits, my lifestyle, etc. I was so excited because I understood what he was saying! I'm a schoolteacher, so I don't consider myself ignorant, but he made health, nutrition, and complex physiology fit together and make sense in a way I had never understood before. I left his office with a sense of purpose, determination, and hope for my future well-being. My journey had begun – and on that day, the numbers on the scale quit climbing.

Nutrition has been the most important factor in my weight loss. I keep a daily food journal that allows me to see in just a glance if my food intake of protein, carbs, and fat is appropriate. I also have managed to work regular exercise into my lifestyle – a feat I had previously claimed was impossible due to lack of valuable time. Joe is always available to me via e-mail for questions, concerns, and most importantly, encouragement. I immediately noticed a huge upsurge in my energy level and that I wasn't experiencing the hunger and mood swings that I had regularly experienced before. I knew in my heart that this time I would succeed!

continued ⟶

Metabolic Transformation in Action

> It wasn't long until friends and family began asking me questions: "You've lost weight! What are you doing?" and "You seem different? What's going on?" It wasn't just the weight they were noticing. It was the difference in my demeanor, attitude, and general outlook on life. My husband and children could see that I was finally returning to the way I used to be – the wife and mom they had been missing so much.
>
> I have tried many, many other weight-loss facilities and programs. They offered counseling sessions, encouraged food journaling, and some even told me exactly what to eat. I managed to lose weight for a while, but something was missing. I always went back to my old habits and gained it back, plus some. After working with Joe, I believe the missing "something" is the fact that he truly cares and believes in you so much, you simply cannot fail! He goes the extra miles it takes to make sure you understand and can succeed. You learn to believe in your own abilities and that translates in to all aspects of your life. When I said life-changing experience at the beginning, I meant life-changing, not just the weight.
>
> As of November 30, 2005 I have lost 54 pounds! I still have a lot of weight to lose, but I have no doubt in my mind that I will lose the weight and keep it off for life. With Dr. Joe's help, I have completely changed my way of thinking about food. In October, my family and I went to Florida for a 10-day vacation and I did not gain an ounce. Believe me, that was a first!
>
> My spiraling journey continues onward and upward now, but the numbers on the scales are going down! Thank you, Dr. Joe! Thank you, Dr. Uloth! I am a different person – the person I need to be for myself and for my family – because you both took the time and effort to care.

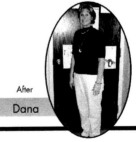

After
Dana

Between meals, body fat is released from body fat cells, but only as much as is needed. So, if you follow the path, this paragraph will be monumental to your understanding. Your food intake is now precise and consistent so that you will get precise and consistent results. The total amount of calories is moderately lower than your body needs on a daily basis so that it requires a secondary source of calories. The first place your body is going to access is blood sugar, liver glycogen, and a moderate amount of available muscle glycogen (especially if you work out).

(Figure 2:5) Step Two

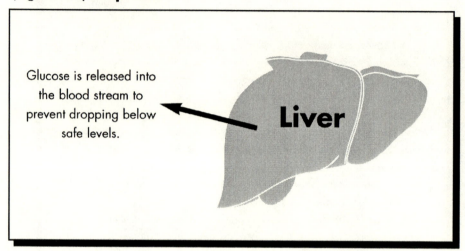

Glucose is released into the blood stream to prevent dropping below safe levels.

Liver

The Diet Docs' Rx chart is designed to take a large portion of the caloric deficit from carbohydrates so that as you continue using blood sugar and glycogen, you will eventually (within two to four days) be as depleted as your brain will safely allow. This is a large portion of the deficit we're creating, but it in no way makes it a low-carbohydrate diet. Blood sugar levels are critical to the brain and body so your brain won't let you go too far without throwing a tantrum. At this point, you'll feel hungry, possibly weak and shaky, maybe tired, and some will even get a headache. Since this is not a low-carb diet, this phase will be brief and is a rite of passage that leads to success. You now have reached a level of carbohydrate depletion that opens a door to significant body-fat loss. If you give in to the hunger at this point, you'll refill your muscle and liver glycogen as well as your blood stream glucose (sugar) and you'll have to *start over*. Unfortunately, this is a pattern of many dieters. Three or four days go well, and then a binge sends them back to the starting block both physically and mentally. What happens in reality is that they deplete and replete carb stores without much alteration in body fat and though they really are eating well 80% of the time, they don't lose weight.

If, however, you stay within your macronutrient range through this tough day of being moderately carb depleted, a great accomplishment takes place.

(Figure 2:6) Final Step in Carb Depletion

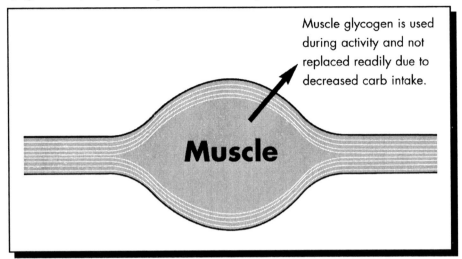

Muscle glycogen is used during activity and not replaced readily due to decreased carb intake.

Since you're not giving in to the carb cravings, your brain is forced into plan B. Plan B is that since you're not providing more glucose from your diet, your body has to find another source. I can't emphasize enough how amazing the design of our body is. Two things will now happen that allows for immediate and consistent body fat loss. Body fat cells start releasing fatty acids and glycerol, the products of stored body fat. Once in the blood stream, some is used directly by certain types of cells for energy (lipolysis) while more actually gets converted into glucose. This mechanism is called gluconeogenesis, literally the creation of new glucose. Now blood sugar levels come back up to a consistent level so energy returns and hunger decreases. As a matter of fact there is almost a euphoric rise in energy and a marked decrease in lethargy throughout the day due to the consistency in blood sugar. This is real energy; not the temporary caffeine or sugar high that leaves you jittery, dazed, and then asleep! As long as you're consistent with your suggested food intake totals, you're now making up the majority of the caloric deficit through the mechanism of turning your body fat into new carbohydrates. It isn't difficult to understand the purpose of this design is so that we can survive for long periods of time by accessing these stored calories in the form of body fat if necessary. By learning how to effectively take advantage of this inherent survival mechanism you're going to lose body fat permanently without the suffering fad diets often cause.

(Figure 2:7) The Breaking Point

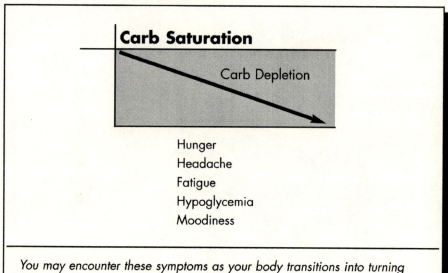

You may encounter these symptoms as your body transitions into turning body fat into glucose but it will be <u>brief</u> because the carb count provided in the Diet Docs' Rx is moderate, not excessively low.

Another way of explaining it is that the brain needs a constant supply of glucose in the blood stream. To make sure glucose levels aren't too high or too low, the brain directs the pancreas to produce more glucagon (to raise blood sugar) or insulin (to store blood sugar). Fat loss or fat gain *isn't* the primary goal of the body with food; it's an indirect effect based on what hormone—glucagon or insulin—is present most often. Too much carbohydrate in one meal results in insulin being dominant and we're in a storage mode. Too little carbohydrate and we're in a retrieving mode. So why not eliminate carbs completely? More on that critical question coming up. When too much carbohydrate is present and insulin runs rampant, we store the glucose in our liver and muscle, (meaning we have to once again deplete that carbohydrate to begin burning body fat maximally), and some of the blood glucose gets directly pulled into fat cells and stored as fat. Note the study regarding yo-yo dieting.

One thing to keep in mind is that each gram of glycogen holds approximately three times its weight in water. A by-product of cellular metabolism is also water. So, the first week of decreasing your body's level of stored carbohydrates and beginning the process of losing body fat will result in a large amount of water loss. It isn't uncommon for someone to lose five to eight pounds in the first week. The second week's weight loss will be a truer reflection of how much body fat is being lost.

Can't I Have Just One Piece of Pizza?

Here's the best news of the book so far. You get a "splurge" meal. Not a splurge day and not a lay-on-the-couch-moaning splurge meal after visiting every buffet in town. If you're on track with your personal Diet Docs' Rx and you're losing at the pace described, you can and should have one meal per week where you enjoy foods you've been avoiding as "not the best weight-loss foods." Have a couple pieces of pizza and a dessert. Have a steak and potato and even a dinner roll. Eat a moderate amount and enjoy it without guilt. You'll be replacing your normal dinner and possibly a snack, so the calorie overage isn't that much; perhaps just barely over your metabolic rate. This does several things. First, you need that boost in food intake so your body doesn't continue in a chronic calorie deficit for too long. Recall the studies showing how fast and how far your metabolism can fall. Secondly, you get a nice break from the deficit and the feeling of being deprived. You may not think you need these breaks. You're tough, right? But chronic depletion can sneak up on you and having this pause only makes you less prone to binging, and as I said, you really do need it physiologically for long-term progress. Some nice side effects are that you get used to eating "normal" or "bad" food, however you want to describe it, without going overboard in volume and you have the flexibility of a floating "meal off" to use for special occasions. Plan your splurge meal for that birthday party or that football game. I would always keep this in play and if it slows your progress down, cut your daily amount of carbs just a little to be able to keep moving forward with the splurge meal.

CHAPTER TWO KEY POINTS

1) Correct nutrition can raise your metabolism to help achieve weight loss.

2) The right amount of food per day is the first and most important step in achieving permanent and predictable weight loss through raising your metabolism.

3) You must follow your macronutrient totals consistently to achieve this predictable body fat loss – take your Rx!

4) It may be necessary to adjust your macronutrient totals.

5) After two to four days, be prepared to feel hungry, tired, and possibly get a headache as your body prepares to begin converting body fat into glucose. Stay on course; it will only last one day at the most.

6) Be patient with the amount of information you are learning. It will continue to make more sense as you keep reading.

CHAPTER THREE

MEAL STRUCTURING—POWER SPACING

Meal Portions

Now that you have established how much food you need per day, how are you to structure this food into your daily meals and snacks? This question is far more important than you might think. You can actually gain or lose weight eating the exact same amount of food just by changing how you schedule your meals during the day.

There is a limit to how much food your body can effectively digest, metabolize, and absorb at one time. If you eat too much at a meal, some of that food ends up stored as new body fat. So even if you're eating the right amount of food per day, you could be working against yourself by storing new body fat at certain meals. At best, this could slow your progress; at worst, it could negate any progress at all. This pattern can result from our culture's typical way of eating: skip breakfast, grab a candy bar or burger at lunch, and then start supper in the kitchen and extend it until bedtime. Recall from chapter two that in creating a calorie deficit we first draw dominantly from intermediate energy, mostly stored glycogen from the liver and muscle. Only when we use most of what is stored there do we switch over in a larger way to stored body fat. If we constantly eat larger meals, even though we stay calorically in line for the day, we have periods of time where we cause insulin to be released in too high of amounts, restore glycogen, and we move out of the accelerated body fat burning mode. Not only does this style of eating promote consuming too much at one time, it also means going for long periods of time without eating. This brings up another problem.

Once digestion, absorption, and metabolism of consumed nutrients have slowed and stopped after a meal, your body starts using stored energy. If you go too long without eating, your metabolic processes taper to conserve energy. So, if you eat only a couple of large meals per day, your body starts converting the excess food from large meals into body fat at the same time that glycogen is being restored. During the long periods between meals, your metabolism slows down. Essentially, you have created a downward spiral of storing new body fat and then made it more difficult to lose due to a slowing metabolism. Furthermore, you will be prone to storing more body fat at the next meal due to the hormonal changes. Talk about a vicious cycle! The act of digesting food and the subsequent increase of cellular metabolism that takes place is actually the greatest way to affect long-term calorie burning. The more times you eat, the higher your metabolism rises within your genetic limit. So, be sure to not skip your snacks.

Skipping a meal or snack once in awhile isn't going to send your metabolism tumbling. Making it a way of life will. The biggest reason that smaller meals work better is so that you don't store extra body fat like you would at larger meals and your metabolism is actually increased every time you eat. If you can raise your metabolism more frequently with smaller meals and you're not storing new fat at those meals, you're in fat-loss overdrive!

Power Spacing

Five to even eight small meals and snacks per day should be a goal. By frequently eating meals small enough so they are completely used and not stored as body fat, you can keep your metabolism charged to maximal levels. Sometimes you may not be hungry for that scheduled snack, but keep your eye on your schedule. If you skip one and then can't eat for another couple of hours, hunger may drive you to binge or eat what you didn't have planned.

Several factors can make it easy to design your meal spacing plan. First and foremost, divide the quantity of macronutrients logically, not necessarily perfectly. Two to three meals per day should be solid, normal meals much the same as you may currently eat, except in the right amounts. (Food choices and actual meals with macronutrient ratios will be discussed in later chapters.) The remaining two to three meals per day will be smaller snacks. Try to eat your meals or snacks every three to four hours. I can hear many of you grumbling, "I don't have time to eat that many times a day!" Scott certainly viewed this as a barrier. Can you imagine being a family practice physician and trying to find time to eat? By 9 in the morning doctors are already 14 hours behind! Be honest, though; we can all sip on a protein shake or stop for five minutes to grab a snack even if we're still working. This is another reason to plan ahead. Power spacing is second only to The Diet Docs' Rx in importance if you want to achieve the safest, most efficient weight loss. This is a difficult, habitual shift for most people, but it is *critical*.

AVERAGE JOE PHYSIOLOGY

The Dynamic Duo – Hormones that is

Believe it or not, gaining or losing body fat is merely a symptom of a delicate balance of hormones in your body. As you now know, insulin causes glucose (carbohydrates) to be stored and glucagon instigates fat loss. Insulin stores; glucagon retrieves. Insulin creates fat stores; glucagon removes stored body fat. In a normal state of balance in the body, three times more insulin is present in the blood stream compared to glucagon. The fact that there is 50 million times greater amounts of blood glucose than these hormones combined, shows how powerful they are in small amounts. Subtle swings in either direction cause major metabolic changes. Consider a visual illustration of a teeter-totter: glucagon on one side, insulin the other. When insulin increases above its normal levels, the body starts storing more energy than normal. If glucagon starts increasing, energy will be harvested within the body. Studies show that when carbohydrates are decreased, glucagon concentration increases. Through a cascade of events, body fat is used as energy as an end result. When meal intervals are well-planned, overt increases in carbohydrates, and therefore insulin, are easier to avoid. Over the course of a day, a week, and a month, one would spend more time with higher blood levels of glucagon compared to insulin and would have lost more body fat even with a similar overall calorie intake. This gives you quite an edge in dieting. You're literally working with your body instead of against it.

Having provided an overview of the importance of meal spacing, I want you to know exactly why this step is so important. Recall from chapter two that your body is essentially in a constant state of metabolic storage or retrieval. Blood nutrient levels are being kept steady by the work of virtually every system of your body. After a meal, the body is working to digest and distribute nutrients in a pattern based on priority. Seemingly frantic processes are occurring to keep the body functioning at its highest level. As those critical needs are being met, however, excess food is quickly stored, since it is not needed at that particular time. Remember, the body is built for survival. What it doesn't need now, it will store to use later. Excess fat in a meal can be stored directly as body fat right out of the bloodstream and excess carbohydrates will be converted into triglycerides and also stuffed into fat cells. Both of these processes will be discussed in depth in upcoming chapters.

(Figure 3:1) Power Spacing

6:00 a.m.	Breakfast
9:00 a.m.	Snack
12:00 p.m.	Lunch
3:00 p.m.	Snack
6:00 p.m.	Supper
9:00 p.m.	Small snack (optional)

The bottom line is that too much food in one meal will create new body fat on the premise that your body will be able to use it later. This happens constantly even to people whose weight is very stable. We store a little body fat and then use it between meals. Those of us that carry more weight than is healthy, though, are walking reminders that we're storing more at those meals than we're ultimately using. The answer isn't to wait longer between meals; the answer is to not overeat at meals and *stop* the storage process before it starts. This is critically important because we store body fat much easier than we use it. Once digestion and absorption are complete after a meal and our blood sugar levels start to lower, we now have to work our way through the newly stored glycogen in the liver and the blood lipids (fat) before we start using a larger portion of stored body fat. If we overeat we may never even get to that level of working our way through our stores before we eat again and restart the process.

Conversely, if we eat meals that contain correct amounts of protein, carbohydrates, and fat to allow our body to function optimally, we increase the likelihood of not storing anything new as fat, and instead spend more time between meals in a retrieval mode of burning stored body fat for energy. You'll find that you're ready for that next meal even if you're not used to eating frequently. You can quickly create a pattern of stability in your metabolism that keeps blood nutrient levels from fluctuating wildly, energy levels high, and body fat usage constant. The alternative of eating larger, less frequent meals will lead to slower weight loss, potential weight gain, and fatigue.

Keep in mind that there really isn't a perfect ratio. I often get asked if meals should be exactly the same size and spaced exactly at certain intervals. If you're that obsessive compulsive, life itself has probably given you an anxiety disorder and I don't want to add to it! It actually is easy to assume that there must be a perfect formula since nutrition is a science, but your daily activity, schedule, and energy expenditure create a ton of metabolic diversity. Depending on your daily living activities and exercise, you may have different metabolic needs and hunger patterns on different days. It's important that you allow yourself the flexibility for your meals to vary in size, time, and content day to day without thinking you're failing. You'll gradually find some habits become mainstays and other meals you may change often. The greatest thing about not being locked into someone else's food plan is that the freedom leads to thinking on your feet. You learn to succeed by using your brain. A novel idea in this era of cookie-cutter diet books!

The Convenience Factor

Eating five to eight times a day poses a scheduling challenge to most people just as it did with Scott. However, just as he discovered, once you have adopted this new way of eating, you will have so much more energy that you'll never want to revert to your past meal pattern. Gone was the temporary, artificial energy brought on by sugar and caffeine, and it was replaced by constant energy from steady blood glucose levels. Eating small, frequent meals keeps nutrients flowing into your body, which is the cornerstone of good health and weight management. Blood sugar, nitrogen (protein), and blood lipid (fat) levels all stay more uniform via small meals. Everyone has experienced lulls (and even crashes) in energy during the day. With well-spaced meals, these lulls will disappear and be replaced with steady, high energy levels.

You can easily overcome meal scheduling challenges with good planning. Meal replacement drinks ("protein shakes") and high-quality food ("energy") bars can be very good, convenient snack choices. Low-glycemic fruit (as discussed in chapter four), yogurt, and many other whole-food choices are also easy to fit into your daily routine. If there is such a thing as meal timing and quantity perfection, you would still have a problem sustaining that "perfect" schedule every day.

The good news is that you don't have to. Some days are understandably going to be wild, on the run, and impossible to do as well as you want. The first thing to always consider is your ultimate goal. If you're in a hurry, don't use it as an excuse to stop for a cookie dough milk shake because you "didn't have time for anything else." It's always better to grab a healthy carb source, like a piece of fruit, even if it causes you to be out of your macronutrient range for the day (because you likely may be low on protein or fat). So the extra carbs won't do that much damage. It may not be a "perfect" day, but it's not a diet catastrophe.

Stay well-armed with good food and plan ahead to make sure you can eat when you should eat, but when all else fails, get the best alternative you can and regroup. This is where your log book comes in handy. If you have a running total of what you've consumed for the day, I guarantee you'll make better choices on the spot. Even with no one looking over your shoulder, it will be rewarding for you to know that you're staying on your plan even in a pinch. These small daily successes will make you a confident weight-loss warrior.

Metabolic Transformation in Action

A few months after I turned 53, I got really tired of the fact that too many of my clothes were fitting tightly, even though I had been jogging, riding my bike, and "watching" what I ate. The weight on my 5'6" frame just seemed to stay around 165 no matter what I did. This was 20 pounds more than I weighed just 10 years earlier. (I had lost 5 pounds on a popular plan when I was 50, but like almost everyone else I know who tried it, I had gained it all back.)

One day I happened to catch Dr. Joe on a local TV show. Having recognized him from church, I called him and set up an hour consultation. Joe's approach to nutrition and good body stewardship has since affected my life very dramatically. In fact, the change has been so dynamic in me, it is a physical equivalent to the spiritual rebirth the Bible speaks of.

Dr. Joe simply gave me an eating plan to make my body start burning stored fat. Within 25 days, I lost 10 pounds of it, and in less than 5 months I was down to 135. My weight has remained between 131 and 135 for 2 years – along with the 30" waist I had in high school!!! My energy and stamina multiplied. I just feel like a new and different person. Medically speaking, my trigycerides have dropped from 249 to 88, my HDL ("good" cholesterol) rose from 46 to 68, and my LDL ("bad" cholesterol) dropped from 122 to 98.

On the Metabolic Transformation plan...
- I did not get the "munchies." I just got hungry for a meal of real food.
- I didn't feel like I was sacrificing anything, food-wise.
- I didn't eat any "weird" food like rice cakes or celery bread or grapefruit rind.
- I was not hungry for the cookies, cake, pie, etc. that had been one of my "basic food groups" all my life. It did not bother me to pass by the many sweets that I frequently encounter during the course of a day.
- I don't have any plan or desire to go back to my old eating habits. I love/enjoy what I am eating now, and could eat this way for the rest of my life.

Part of Joe's strategy is strengthening the body through weight training. This has been extremely invigorating. With the newfound energy that intelligent eating gives me, I am able to do a vigorous work out 3 times a week, and so at 55 am in the best shape of my life! Last year I set personal

continued ⟶

Metabolic Transformation in Action

lifetime speed records for running the 5K, and was also able to climb 5,235 feet to the ridge crest of Mt. Whitney (13,600 ft) and back in one day.

I have come to realize that an hour of vigorous exercise is NOT a waste of time "when you should be doing something more important." It is tuning up your body so you can accomplish in a more efficient way what God needs you to. The hour I spend lifting weights or running I get back in the one less hour of sleep I need, a more alert mind, and relaxed body.

I know that there are many weight-loss theories and programs; however, I can't help thinking there is something very unique and permanent about Metabolic Transformation. And you won't find anyone with a keener mind who is more concerned about your total well being than Dr. Joe. The surge in my self-confidence that he gave me has resulted in positive effects too numerous to mention. Thanks a million, Joe!

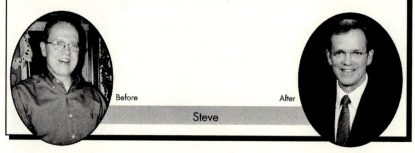

Before — Steve — After

CHAPTER THREE KEY POINTS

• • • ▶ 1) Too much food at one meal leads to new body fat storage.

• • • ▶ 2) Too much time between meals slows the metabolism.

• • • ▶ 3) Five to seven small meals/snacks can maximize metabolic rate and keep body fat loss consistent.

• • • ▶ 4) Well-planned and spaced meals will lead to steady, high energy levels throughout the entire day.

• • • ▶ 5) Convenience is very important. Plan ahead to make sure you can eat when you should.

• • • ▶ 6) An ounce of preparation is worth a pound on your waistline.

CHAPTER FOUR

CARBOHYDRATES: THEY'RE NOT JUST FOR BREAKFAST ANYMORE

Friend or Foe?

Chapters two and three answered structural questions: how much should I eat, and how should I create and space my meals? Now the discussion moves directly to food. As discussed previously, food is divided into three main macronutrients: protein, carbohydrates, and fat. Each is dramatically different both in structure and function. A calorie isn't just a calorie. A calorie is a unit of energy, a measurement. One gram of carbohydrate equals four calories as does one gram of protein. Fat, often called a more "dense" nutrient, has nine calories per gram. Even though each calorie is the same unit of energy, the effect on your body's chemistry and function is quite different depending on its source (protein, carbs, or fat). That is why some methods of weight loss are more effective than others. Each macronutrient will be covered in its own chapter. We begin with the most controversial.

Many dietitians and nutritionists have elevated carbohydrates to an almost untouchable level of nutritional deity. For decades, dieticians devised weight-loss schemes with carbohydrates at the center of the diets. Until recently, commercials bragged about how cereals are full of "nutritious carbohydrates." Witness now everyone's change in language to "whole grains" since the low-carb craze has made "carbohydrate" a dirty word. One problem is that processed white flour isn't a whole grain.

Long before nutrition was a studied science, it was understood that athletes needed more fuel—more calories—to support their training. Like now, carbohydrates were the most abundant, least expensive, most convenient, and usually best-tasting food. Since athletes were observed consuming many more carbohydrates than anyone else and had physiques that were admired by all, the conclusion was drawn that eating carbs was the way to go. My more science-oriented readers (like my organic chemistry professor who stained my transcript with the only "C" that appears in over 10 years of college meandering—I still haven't forgiven him), may already be able to conclude that correlation does not equal causation. Athletes may be able to eat a great deal of carbohydrates and not gain body fat due to their intense levels of training, but what about those of us who don't train as hard? And just because athletes may "get away" with eating too many carbs because of their energy expenditure, does that mean it's the best nutrition even for them?

AVERAGE JOE PHYSIOLOGY

> ### Double Your Fat Loss
>
> *In a review of isocaloric diet studies (diets that compare the same amount of calories but with different ratios of protein, carbohydrates, and fat) it is difficult to find outcomes different than was found by the International Journal of Obesity. Studies were reviewed and compared that controlled subject group calories at 1,000 and were divided into higher-carbohydrate/low-fat groups and higher-fat/low-carbohydrate groups. Other studies were reviewed using the same type of nutrient ratios but even higher calories. The groups on lower carbohydrates, but the same amount of overall calories, lost 43% more weight. That is a strong indictment against high-carb diets, but not necessarily an endorsement of no-carb diets. As you will see, carbs have their place and taking their elimination to an extreme will cause extreme problems. Carbohydrates are a key variable, but knowing what the correct level to decrease them to depends on several factors.*

Of course, the inevitable response to one extreme is always the opposite extreme, so it didn't take long for no-carbohydrate diets to creep onto the scene like a brain fog. To answer these questions and cut our way through a still raging controversy, let's turn to metabolic physiology. (Or, if I've lost you already, take a break and turn to the sports page or the comics for awhile and then come back. I'll wait.) Once you understand exactly what happens inside your body when you eat different foods, you will be able to discern good nutrition from bad.

(Figure 4:1) Carbohydrate Digestion

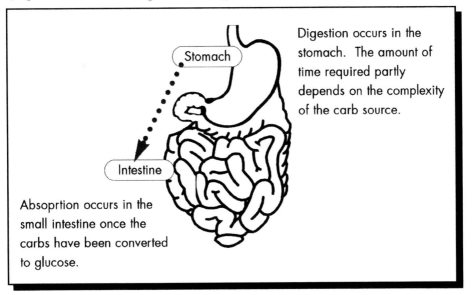

Digestion occurs in the stomach. The amount of time required partly depends on the complexity of the carb source.

Absoprtion occurs in the small intestine once the carbs have been converted to glucose.

Carbohydrate Structure and Function

Carbohydrates provide most of the energy for our bodies most of the time. Because they require the least amount of energy to break down, carbohydrates are the easiest of the macronutrients to digest and be converted to glucose. Carb sources are loosely described as sugars, starches, or fibers, and these are commonly described as simple and complex carbohydrates. We typically think of simple carbohydrates as junk food, like soda and candy, and complex carbs as whole foods, like potatoes, pasta, and bread. This type of categorization leads to the false assumption that a particular food is either good or bad when actually there is more of a continuum that allows detailed comparison. Good, better, best, bad, and/or worse may be more appropriate ways of describing carb choices once you understand how they compare to one another and how they affect your body. (Didn't Jerry Springer do a show on this: bad carbs and the women who love them?)

Glucose is the smallest sugar molecule possible. It is the form of sugar that the human body uses for energy. Whatever form of carbohydrate you consume, the end result of digestion is glucose. There are, however, many forms of carbohydrates, and the pathway of digestion that leads to glucose is what can affect our energy levels, mental acuity, physical functioning, and even athletic performance.

You may recognize the names of various forms of sugar: glucose, lactose, fructose, maltose, dextrose, sucrose, and so on. Each one of these carbohydrates has a different level of molecular complexity. Those that are made primarily of glucose are easy and quick to digest since most of the carbs are already in the smallest possible form. (For dieters, that's bad.) Those with a more complex molecular structure are harder to digest and take longer to move through the digestion process. (That's good!) The *Glycemic Index* (Fig. 4:8) is a scale that ranks carbohydrate foods by comparing their structures. It reveals the simplicity or complexity of the sugar, starch, and fiber that make up the macronutrient called carbohydrates.

(Figure 4:2) Insulin Reaction

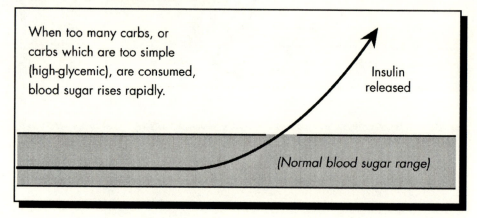

Just to Make Sure You're Still Awake

Two caveats that need explanation are fiber and sugar alcohols. The popularity of low-carb diets have led people to believe that fiber and sugar alcohol is "free" and doesn't need counted. Fiber, though it is digested slower, is a carbohydrate. Any that doesn't get digested in the stomach can be actually broken down in the large intestine. So, while fibrous carbs are good, healthy sources, they are still, and must be counted as, carbohydrates.

An interesting carbohydrate source that the FDA hasn't classified firmly (gee, the government confusing us? Who'd of thought?) is sugar alcohol, or polyphenols. Used in some baked products, and very prevalent in protein/energy bars, sugar alcohol (usually in the form of glycerine or glycerol) is actually part of a fat molecule. Being calorically similar to a carbohydrate, but structurally coming from a fat molecule, and the fact that it is digested very slowly without a fast rise in blood sugar (did I mention this was confusing?) originally led the FDA to not even require listing it on the label. Talk about denial—we don't know what it is, so we'll just ignore it? Whether due to lobbying efforts by the low-carb food producers or due to the reduced danger to diabetics (since it doesn't cause a fast rise in blood sugar) sugar alcohol was allowed to fly under the radar. When the outcry was loud enough, the FDA started requiring them to be rightly listed in "total carbohydrates" on the label, but they continue to allow fiber and polyphenols to be deducted to create a new category: net carbs. Again, these carbs are there and need to be counted. Don't deduct fiber and ignore "net carb" counts; track "total carbohydrates."

Alcoholic beverages are similar but don't even (as of yet) provide the courtesy of the "net carb" label. Look at any low-carb, light beer and you'll find near-zero protein and fat counts, a low carbohydrate count, but calories listed at a much higher level than if you did the math. (Protein and carbs have four calories per gram and fat has nine.) The "missing calories" are carbs not counted—sugar alcohol. Wine and hard liquor are roughly four grams of carbs per ounce, though they'll be often listed as just one. Those light beers that you think you've been downing at a cost of only 7 to 10 grams of carbs are really about 20 to 25. (Sheesh!!! These Diet Docs are no fun—as a matter of fact, forget it; I'm going onto the next bestseller that plays along and lets me drink beer! And, while I'm at it, I'm going to eat all the chips and pretzels I want too; so there!!)

Back to Business

When you consume a high-glycemic index carbohydrate such as white bread, a banana, a baked potato, soda, candy, etc., you are consuming a carbohydrate that is primarily glucose. Little digestion needs to take place with these foods. They pass through the stomach quickly and enter the small intestine. Absorption occurs in the small intestine, and since so much glucose enters so fast, uptake is rapid. Your brain closely monitors your blood sugar levels, and such a rapid increase triggers your pancreas to release the hormone insulin. Remember, insulin is the storage hormone that shuttles blood glucose where it is needed.

Most of us aren't glycogen-depleted (short of stored glucose), so our muscles and livers usually contain *plenty* of glucose for fuel. Depending on how many carbohydrates you consume at one time, chances are you will have too much blood sugar and nowhere to store it. Your already high level of circulating insulin causes your liver to convert the blood sugar into triglycerides (fat) to be ultimately stored. Insulin also triggers body fat cells to simply pull excess glucose in to be converted directly into body fat.

(Figure 4:3) Carbohydrate Conversion to Body Fat

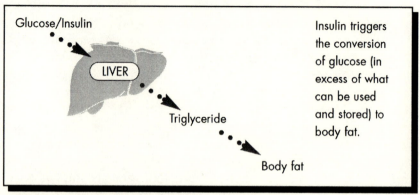

None of the aforementioned high-glycemic carb sources have fat in them, but a large portion of the carbs can be converted to body fat due to the effect of insulin. Unfortunately, the problems don't stop there. Be it by storage, utilization, or by fat conversion, your blood glucose levels return to normal and your brain tells your pancreas to stop releasing insulin. However, even with the process stopped, a certain amount of insulin remains active in the bloodstream until it is "used up." This means more blood sugar will be removed, dropping it below the normal level. A blood sugar level that's too low will leave you tired as in the case of the after-lunch dosing behind the desk. Even worse, your brain sends out powerful hormonal messengers to signal hunger. I'm sure you've experienced eating something and being even hungrier a short while later. Too much of a drop and you can have more severe symptoms such as hypoglyecemia. Have you ever ended up weak, shaky, and starving just 30 or 60 minutes after eating?

(Figure 4:4) Insulin Overcompensation

The tragedy of this whole process is it takes you from bad to worse in body composition, energy levels, and health in one fell swoop. You either block body fat loss or store new body fat with a "fat-free" food. You then end up tired and so hungry with carbohydrate cravings that you eat a similar meal and start the process all over again. This is an extremely powerful biochemical reaction. Massive, seemingly uncontrollable binges are birthed by insulin-induced low blood sugar. Many of us live on this roller coaster and don't realize that we're the ones causing it! "I just have a slow metabolism," or "You just naturally gain more body fat as you get older . . ."—I know you've used these excuses, and I know you've believed them. It's time to gain control over your nutrition for good.

Falling Off the Wagon

Binging isn't an eating disorder, though it can lead to one. Binging is often rooted in the physiology of dieting too hard. When you sustain too low of a carbohydrate level for too long, your body is going to crave carbs and most of us aren't going to be able to stop eating once we start. It's common but it's devastating. Listen in to an e-mail from a client:

> *"So . . . I knew it would not take long before you discovered the real me. I haven't sent you this week's food diary but suffice it to say that it is not good at all. This is me. Unable to stick to clean eating for more than days at a time, disgusted with myself, and firmly believing that it is my destiny to be chubby and miserable all the time. Yet I make these choices. I understand that each time I eat ice cream or chocolate or whatever, that I am making the choice to do so. What I don't know is why I can't seem to correct my behavior. And I don't consider myself one of those people who cheats just to try to get away with as much as possible. No, I try, oh, Lord, how I do try . . . then I crack and I eat something I shouldn't because I just HAVE TO . . . then I can't stop so I eat more. Then I feel guilty and disgusted with myself. Then I get into a cycle o,f 'Well, you've already screwed up so if you do it again it doesn't matter.' And I do, which perpetuates the cycle. Then I get really mad at myself and say, 'Okay, get over it, move on, you'll be okay.' And I go great guns and do really well until yet again, after days of pacing around my kitchen looking at food or gazing at the giant cookies at the supermarket, I give in and the self-destruction begins again. 'Well, I screwed up and ate the cookies so if I eat this cake too it doesn't matter.' It doesn't seem to matter how much variation I get, how many carbs or how little, there is stuff I WANT and I can never seem to shake it. And it's very bad when I am at work with all the treats people bring in. I know my choices only hurt my chances*

of achieving my goal, yet I do it any way. Through weeks and weeks of dieting I tell myself how much I am sacrificing and suffering and I think, 'Why go through all of this and then mess it up for a piece of pie?' But somehow I manage (in the moment) to justify that it won't matter. Am I insane? Am I just a loser?"

Have you been there? I have. Scott has. He would say that if he didn't drink any soda he would be fine, but if he had one before the end of the day, it would turn into three. There are three critical points I want you to see illustrated in that e-mail. The first is the cycle I mentioned above: if you don't give yourself a chance to move away from the dominance of over-consuming carbohydrates, and if you never get past that "sticking point" and make it into a couple of days of stability, you may stay in that miserable cycle. The second point is that it does take a few days for your body to stabilize and it DOES get easier. Hunger decreases, cravings decrease, and it's a very noticeable shift. Both of these points are physical. It is sugar withdrawal, and you have to get through it. These biological impulses are going to happen regardless of how strong—or weak-willed you may be in the moment of temptation. Power spacing will help you get through this detox—use it. The last point, though, is your will. During those tough points, it helps to have a sense of righteous indignation—"I'm not putting THAT in my body!" Or a sense of mission and pride—"Being lean means more to me than that cookie! I can do it!!" Avoid having those foods around, ask those around you to help, do anything you think will help, but get beyond this roller coaster and make it easier for yourself. Once you move into a deeper level of body fat metabolism through controlled and consistent carbohydrate intake, stability will be just around the corner.

Stability Can Be Controlled; by You!

Now that you actually *understand* the physiological problems created by getting outside your ranges (getting too high and spiking your insulin thereby causing fat storage, or getting too low and setting off a hypoglycemic eating binge) you can move to *permanent* control. You are not a "loser" and you are not "insane," but don't do the "whatever" eating and quit doing "I've already screwed up so I might as well keep going." Those behaviors only lead to greater fat storage. If you must have a treat, don't view yourself as a failure. Everyone loves a treat. I know I sure as heck do! Simply try to make better choices for that treat. Eat in control, keep close to your ranges, and you'll be fine. You are well on your way to understanding and working smarter not harder. Quit putting yourself in a shame spiral and beating yourself up. You *can* do this. I will further caution you to not let sugary treats become a habit and replace a large portion of your carbohydrate ranges. You might be able to fit 46 grams of carbs from a soda into your daily ranges, but you will be crowding out healthy carb sources such as fruits, vegetables, and whole grains in addition to harming your pancreas and making your body work harder to lose weight. Don't do it. Concentrate on health and the things that will make it easier to succeed.

What if you chose a carbohydrate on the other end of the glycemic index, such as a grapefruit, an apple, a bowl of oatmeal, or even a salad? These carb sources have different molecular configurations of glucose. Fructose, cellulose, galactose, etc., are much more complex forms of carbohydrate. When these hit your stomach, digestion takes longer to break them into usable glucose molecules. Since this process takes more time, the molecules enter the small intestine and are absorbed more gradually. Blood sugar levels now rise more slowly, avoiding a major insulin increase. Just by changing the carb source you have decreased the potential for the creation of new body fat, and your energy level rises over the next couple of hours instead of plummeting quickly. Possibly best of all for someone who is dieting, hunger is dramatically reduced because blood glucose levels are stable instead of too low, such as at the end of an insulin rampage.

(Figure 4:5) Stable Blood Sugar Through Carbohydrate Management

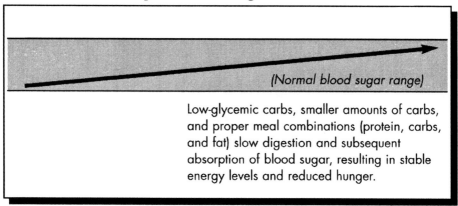

(Normal blood sugar range)

Low-glycemic carbs, smaller amounts of carbs, and proper meal combinations (protein, carbs, and fat) slow digestion and subsequent absorption of blood sugar, resulting in stable energy levels and reduced hunger.

Think back to our chapter two discussion of the opposite effects of insulin and glucagon. During a new client consultation just last week, my new "student" said, "So keeping insulin low is the whole key?" Though there are so many swirling factors occurring at once and so many things depend on one another or affect each other, I had to simply admit, "Yes." Insulin and glucagon are the two opposing hormones that keep blood sugar either increasing or decreasing to normal levels. If we need more glucose, glucagon is produced and through all the complex machinations discussed, we end up losing fat. When there is excess glucose, insulin is produced to bring blood sugar down and part or most of it is stored as fat. We're either storing or retrieving.

(Figure 4:6) The Energy Continuum

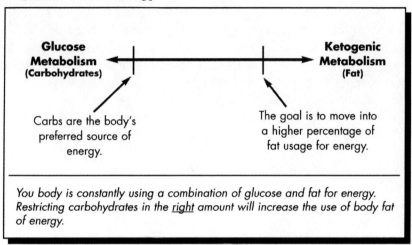

You body is constantly using a combination of glucose and fat for energy. Restricting carbohydrates in the _right_ amount will increase the use of body fat of energy.

When carbs are eaten in the smaller and appropriate amounts, in your personal Rx, insulin is held at bay and glucagon is present more often and in higher amounts and voila: body fat loss. An oversimplified explanation, but it is the "whole key."

(Figure 4:7) Work with Your Body

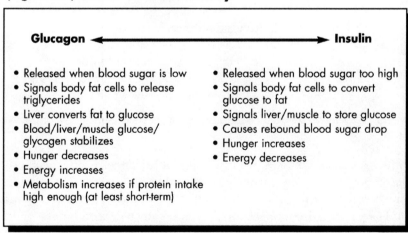

(Figure 4:8) Sample Glycemic Index Selections

The glycemic index essentially rates the speed of digestion of carbohydrates and thus the impact on blood sugar elevation. A zero rating could indicate no carbohydrates present, glucose is rated at a value of 100, and very simple carbohydrates can reach a value much higher than 100.

	Glycemic Index Value	Serving Size	Grams of Carbs per Serving
CEREALS AND BREADS			
All Bran®	30	1/2 cup	15
Oatmeal (rolled oats)	42	1/2 cup (dry)	27
Oatbran bread	47	1 slice	18
Rye bread	58	1 slice	14
Raisin Bran™	61	1/2 cup	19
Pancakes	67	2-4"	58
Special K™	69	1 cup	21
Bagel, white	72	1	70
Grape Nuts™	75	1/4 cup	22
Shredded Wheat™	75	1 cup	30
English muffin	77	1	14
Whole wheat bread	77	1 slice	12
White bread	80	1 slice	14
Crispix™	87	1 cup	25
Rice Krispies™	87	1 cup	21
Corn Flakes™	92	1 cup	26
SNACKS			
Potato chips	57	2 oz	18
Blueberry muffin	59	3.5 oz	47
Tortilla chips	63	2 oz	30
MET-Rx Bar®	74	3.6 oz	50
Soda crackers	74	5	15
Rice cake	82	1	7
Pretzels	83	1 oz	20

	Glycemic Index Value	Serving Size	Grams of Carbs per Serving
COMMON "STARCH" SOURCES FOR MEALS			
Pasta, wheat	32	1 cup	32
Pasta, white	38	1 cup	32
Sweet potato	44	5 oz	25
Rice, brown	50	1/2 cup	17
Rice, long-grain	61	1/2 cup	18
Rice, white	87	1/2 cup	28
Potato, baked	85	5 oz	30
FRUIT			
Cherries	22	1/2 cup	10
Grapefruit	25	1/2	11
Apple	38	4 oz	15
Pear	38	4 oz	11
Orange	42	4 oz	11
Peach	42	4 oz	11
Grapes	46	1 cup	24
Banana	52	4 oz	24
Raisins	64	1/2 cup	44
Cantaloupe	65	4 oz	6
Pineapple	66	4 oz	10
Watermelon	72	4 oz	6
VEGETABLES			
Broccoli	15	1 cup	5
Cauliflower	15	1 cup	5
Lettuce	15	1 cup	2
Carrots	47	1 cup	10
Peas	48	1/2 cup	10
Corn	60	1/2 cup	18

(The New Glucose Revolution, by Jennie Brand-Miller is recommended for further values and understanding of the glycemic index.)

Meal Combinations

The glycemic index is extremely important to your dieting success. Some "nutritionists" don't place much value on this tool, and some act like it doesn't even exist. Yet it can be your greatest asset or your greatest enemy. Many individuals have enjoyed early dieting success with faultless nutrition and then have unknowingly eaten a high-glycemic carb only to be slammed with raging hunger and an insulin-induced tailspin. I think we've all been there—four or five days into a "diet," we find ourselves at the bottom of a gallon of ice cream or lying on the couch with our pants unsnapped after an extended visit to the all-you-can-eat buffet! Now that we know what causes that behavior, we won't let it happen again. The same thing can occur, though, if we go too low on carbohydrates for too long. Anyone who has followed their peers over the low-carb diet cliff knows that powerful hormonal cravings are unleashed that even the strongest-willed can't withstand. Both missteps lead to the same demise. A badly-timed high-glycemic carb or going too long without carbohydrates can lead to low enough blood sugar levels that you suffer with unnecessary hunger, an energy crash, or a head-first dive into a binge.

(Figure 4:9) Sugar Saving Substitutions

Several sugar substitutes exist and may be used to replace sugar sources in cooking, baking, and general sweetening. Though tastes are individual, most artificial sweetener packets can replace two teaspoons of sugar. Non-calorie sweeteners include stevia, aspartame (Equal®), saccharin (Sweet 'N Low®), acesulfame K, and sucralose (Splenda®). My recommendation is stevia, an almost non-caloric sweetening agent derived from a cactus-like plant.

Sugar	Substitutes (packets)	Substitutes (bulk)
2 teaspoons	1 packet	1/2 teaspoon
1/4 cup	6 packets	3 teaspoons
1/3 cup	8 packets	4 teaspoons
1/2 cup	12 packets	6 teaspoons
3/4 cup	18 packets	9 teaspoons
1 cup	24 packets	12 teaspoons

Your own gastrointestinal system actually gives you a carbohydrate safety net, if you know how to use it properly. So far, I've given examples of low—and high-glycemic carb digestive pathways. The glycemic index is a continuum, however, and every food fits in somewhere. Obviously, staying as low as possible will offer the best results with the least "discomfort," but what if you *really* want a carb source that's not as low on the index as you wish it was? Protein and fat molecules are larger and denser than carbohydrates, and digesting them takes between one and three hours, sometimes longer. The valve (pyloric sphincter) between the stomach and small intestine will stay closed as digestion takes place, opening only one to three times per minute while the food is broken down. If you eat a carb source in combination with fat and protein, the carbohydrate gets caught up in the slowed digestive process. In short, a carb eaten alone will be digested and absorbed much faster than one eaten with fat and protein. Remember, slowed absorption of our carbs is a very good thing! Keep in mind that we want to emphasize the practical side of nutrition as well. Don't misunderstand and think that every meal or snack has to have a "perfect" balance of nutrients or that you can never eat a carbohydrate food alone. Between meals that contain good amounts of protein, sometimes a stand-alone carb is a great snack especially something healthy and low-glycemic like a piece of fruit or vegetables.

CHAPTER FOUR KEY POINTS

1) *Carbohydrates provide your body's primary source of energy. Limiting carbohydrates forces the body to use an alternative energy source: body fat.*

2) *High-glycemic carbs promote body fat creation, increased hunger, and decreased energy.*

3) *Low-glycemic carbs increase energy, decrease hunger, and help to avoid body fat storage as opposed to high-glycemic carbs.*

4) *Combining carbs with fat and protein further slows absorption of carbohydrates (refer to later chapter on Meal Planning).*

CHAPTER FIVE

THE SKINNY ON FAT

The Great Myth

"Eat anything you want as long as you don't eat fat." Have you heard people say such a thing? This has been an accepted "fact" for a long time—until recently that is. You will still find these ideas printed in nutrition textbooks, but we're two fad-diet-generations beyond counting fat grams. We've gone from patting every drop of fat from a chicken breast to painstakingly portioning every bite of food into a perfect balance to eating bacon, burgers, and butter, and now it's time to explain which end is up in all of this mayhem. You now know that carbohydrates are physiologically and practically the most important component in fat loss. But dietary fat comes in a close second and actually works hand-in-hand with carbs. As a matter of fact, a physiology professor of mine was fond of the saying, "Fat is burned in the flames of carbohydrates." You have to have a certain amount of carbohydrates to keep your metabolism normal so you can actually burn body fat. The metabolism of fat, though, comes with even more misconceptions and misinformation. Fat and carbohydrate intake and their effect on weight loss are very intertwined.

There are two main divisions of dietary fat: saturated and unsaturated. Saturated fats most commonly come from animal sources. Beef, pork, dairy products, eggs, and poultry contain saturated fats. Products made with these animal fats—such as butter, cream, and many others—are also saturated. Some choices obviously have a great deal more or less fat than others. For example, fish, chicken, and turkey breast have dramatically less than does beef.

The problems with saturated fats lie primarily in their structure. They are much larger and more stable than unsaturated fats and therefore much harder to break down. Since they don't break down easily, they circulate in the blood stream longer, create higher blood cholesterol levels, lead to atherosclerosis, and much of it ends up being stored as body fat. There really aren't many positive things to say about saturated fats. You've undoubtedly heard the term "trans-fat." A fat can be classified either as a cis—or a trans-fat depending on its chemical structure. Trans-fats in general are those that are solid at room temperature and used in junk food and cheap food processing. Your cell membranes are made up of fat molecules that create receptor sites, like "ports," for certain chemicals like glucose, to be shuttled inside the cell. Trans-fats are rotated and stuck in a "backward" position that doesn't allow this to happen, so the cell can't function properly. Trans-fats have been linked to cancer as well as heart disease (as with any saturated fat).

Unsaturated fats are found mainly in plant sources such as olive oil, canola oil, flaxseed oil, grapeseed oil, borage oil, some nuts, and actually in some fish like salmon. Molecularly, unsaturated fats are smaller, less stable, and easier to break down. Surprisingly, unsaturated fats actually have some important health benefits and can help you lose body fat! Many unsaturated fats contain certain specific "essential fatty acids." Each essential fatty acid has unique properties and benefits to the human body. (Notice they're called "essential," a biological term meaning your body can't produce them so you need to supply them.)

Good Fat?

Most people have heard the terms "good fat" and "bad fat." I can assure you that without some unsaturated dietary fat, body fat loss will be slow at first, minimal at best, and ultimately counterproductive. Let me explain these claims. Some essential fatty acids are the building blocks for certain hormones that control fat loss and storage and the potential for muscle gain and loss. Reread that sentence. One more time, please . . . Yes, your body produces specific hormones that control how much body fat you can lose or gain and how much muscle you can gain or lose. Your body needs unsaturated fats (essential fatty acids) to create many of these hormones such as testosterone. In a matter of weeks, people who consume a no—or low-fat diet start producing less and less of the "good" hormones that promote body fat loss and muscle gain. Conversely, people who consume 20 to 30% of their calories from unsaturated fat start producing more of these hormones, often above normal levels. With an increase in your hormonal base, you can actually burn more body fat than normal and build more muscle than normal. Research has demonstrated these incredibly positive blood chemistry changes can lead to decreased cholesterol and increased athletic performance. A little of the *right* dietary fat goes a long way.

(Figure 5:1) Hormones

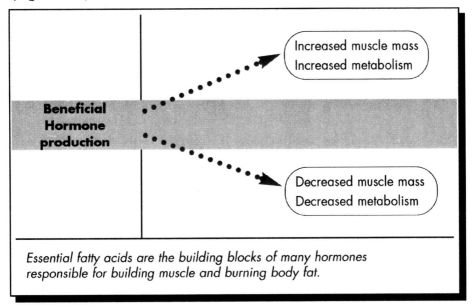

Essential fatty acids are the building blocks of many hormones responsible for building muscle and burning body fat.

I have personally witnessed dramatic decreases in cholesterol and LDL's (low-density lipoproteins, or "bad fat" in the bloodstream) by increasing total dietary fat. I have to qualify this, however, with what I see as a very practical aspect of body fat loss and dieting. Most people who are over weight and eating a poor diet often consume too much refined carbohydrate and too much saturated fat. A few hold-overs from the low-fat craze are eating healthy and fall into the category of "need more good fat," but most of us—whether we care to admit it or not—are killing ourselves on both ends. Therefore, switching to 20 to 30% of calories coming from good fat may cause an overall reduction in body fat. You achieve the best health and best results by eliminating saturated fats and increasing unsaturated fats while keeping carbs in check. You can't leave out carbohydrate control when discussing cholesterol.

Up to 80% of your body's cholesterol is produced in your liver as a result of sugar and runaway insulin. Recall from chapter four that excess carbohydrates result in a conversion to cholesterol and fat. By recommending higher intake of unsaturated fats while controlling carbohydrate levels, I have witnessed hypercholesterolemic clients (those whose livers produce a significantly larger amount of cholesterol) lower their cholesterol levels and manage them so well that, under the supervision of their physicians, they have been able to eliminate the use of cholesterol-reducing medications. A patient referred to me decreased his blood triglycerides from over 900 to 90 in 3 months using the *Metabolic Transformation* program along with weight training and cardiovascular exercise. A triglyceride level of 900! His poor heart was pumping pudding, not blood! Diet should be the cornerstone of any cholesterol management program, not an afterthought. If you need medication, then take it; heart disease is serious business. However, cholesterol-lowering medication shouldn't be viewed as the cure or an excuse to not lose weight and exercise.

(Figure 5:2) Good Fats/Bad Fats

Unsaturated Fats:	Saturated Fats:
*Easily used as energy	*Difficult to breakdown
*Decrease cholesterol	*Increase cholesterol
*Contain essential fatty acids	
*Necessary for many regenerative body processes	
*Necessary to create certain hormones for optimal health, building muscle, and burning body fat	

Another practical example of the power of correct nutrition is seen in elite athletes whose body composition changes are easily measured and observed. I have personally consulted with and supervised the nutrition of hundreds of bodybuilders preparing for competition. They often need to lose between 15 and 40 pounds of body fat for the contest without losing muscle, and this can certainly be achieved. However, I have also tested the body composition of competitors who were not receiving proper nutritional support, and I have been amazed at how much muscle can be lost during dieting; quite a contrast to physiologically sound nutrition.

Burgers and Oils

Consciously switching from saturated to unsaturated fat is a lot easier on paper than it is in real life. You can switch from a hamburger to a chicken breast, or from three whole eggs to six egg whites, but how are you going to get the good fat into your day? The most practical and healthy ways will be to add certain oils to your food. Over time you will naturally start making better food choices and become more creative. For example, if you have a bowl of oatmeal, add one half to a whole tablespoon of flaxseed oil after it's cooked. Do the same thing with brown rice, yogurt, protein shakes, or anything else that can withstand oil without destroying the taste of the food.

If you're making an egg white omelet, cook it with olive, canola, or grapeseed oil instead of a spray. If salad dressing is an area from which you get some of your fat intake, use an Italian dressing made with olive oil instead of a cream-based dressing with saturated fat. Almonds are a very healthy fat source that is very practical for a snack. Watch your serving size; one can is *not* a serving. Be patient and make the process fun, not overwhelming.

I'm tempted to just leave it at avoiding saturated fat; that would be easier. Adding good fat can be another detail that complicates the process, but essential fatty acids must be integrated into your diet for all of the reasons discussed above. They are necessary for your long-term health, for reducing cholesterol, and for creating hormones. Furthermore, a well-placed snack that contains these concentrated healthy fats will sustain energy and decrease hunger longer. They can put the power in power spacing!

A Little More Detail

A point that must be understood is how dynamic fat is in the body. If you gained 10 pounds last year, you're not retaining the exact same 10 pounds of body fat that was originally stored. Your body is constantly storing triglycerides in adipose (fat) cells and also releasing them as you need more energy between meals. In fact, adipose cells always store fat after meals and then release it when needed. Fat is actually used for up to 60% of the body's energy needs at rest A surprising point to most is how easily your body stores dietary fat as body fat. Dietary fat is the easiest nutrient for your body to store as body fat, which makes sense when you think about it. As digested dietary fat is carried past adipose cells in the bloodstream through capillaries, adipose cells simply intake the fat to be stored. As a matter of fact, when you eat just 3% more calories than your body needs at one time, dietary fat is going to be stored in this manner. It takes 25% more food than your body needs at one time to start converting excess carbohydrates into body fat. I know that may sound contradictory as we have made such a big deal of carbohydrates, but don't throw the baby out with the bath water. It is a fact that dietary fat is easier to store as body fat than carbohydrates when calorie intake is more than your body can digest and use at that particular meal. Carbohydrate sources have to be digested, converted into smaller saccharides, dismantled, and then reassembled into fatty acid chains in order to be converted to storable body fat. You need to keep carbs lower and in control to get to the exceptionally accelerated fat loss potential described in chapter one, but you have to keep everything in perspective. Food volume (The Diet Docs' Rx) is step one, power spacing is step two, carb quality and quantity is step three, and then fat closely follows in importance.

Metabolic Transformation in Action

What a blessing it's been to learn about life-changing nutrition from Joe Klemczewski! There aren't enough superlatives to describe him and his vast knowledge of nutrition and the human body. He genuinely cares about teaching people how to eat so our bodies can be as strong and healthy as God created them to be.

I had been active all my life in many different sports. I excelled in dance (mainly ballet), swimming, aerobics, and karate. I never had to worry about what or how much I ate. It did not affect my weight.

In 1992 my food habits changed. I was eating out a lot and eating more of everything, especially sweets. I had moved to a new city and most of my athletic activities stopped. I jumped five sizes as my weight climbed. I had to do something. I altered what I was eating and started riding my bike and walking. Unfortunately, it wasn't working. My weight increased even more.

For a Christmas gift in 1999 my daughters gave me a gift certificate to Joe's gym. He suggested an appointment to talk about nutrition. Joe taught me that the body needs certain amounts of protein, carbohydrates, and good fat. I also learned I needed to eat six or seven times a day, maintaining these certain amounts that he suggested based on my body size and activity level. I wish anyone with a weight issue could learn what I did from Joe. The results will be good health and body leanness that can be enjoyed for the rest of life.

Because I followed Joe's plan, I immediately started losing weight. In just three months my weight was back where I wanted it. I was gaining muscle and had more energy. I was getting stronger and it felt great. With the weight under control and a commitment to continue exercising, I was able to maintain this accomplishment.

Looking back at those first days in the gym, I was so self-conscious of my legs rubbing together I would wear sweats to hide my legs and, yes, a tee shirt to hide the flab on my arms. Once I lost the weight I timidly wore workout shorts and a workout top in the gym. Someone said, "Tootie, where have you been hiding those muscles?!" Wow! What a mental boost! I felt like I had really accomplished something. That was the end of the cover-me-up clothes! It was the turning point in my training.

Joe made me feel like I was the only client he had. Taking a genuine interest in people, their accomplishments, and helping them achieve their goals, Joe is right there to take you to your maximum potential. After being

continued ⟶

Metabolic Transformation in Action

> exposed to some people in the gym and watching how hard they work to compete in bodybuilding and admiring their chiseled bodies, I set a never-before-imagined goal of doing the same.
>
> This was something that I would love to have done in my twenties. Was it possible to do now at age 61? After talking to Joe, it was agreed. I would compete in the 2001 INBF Mid-America Muscle Classic Women's Grand Masters.
>
> I was excited, a little nervous (actually petrified describes it best), but definitely determined. My training became more intense as did my determination. Besides lifting weights, we put a lot of time into selecting music, choreographing a routine, and practicing posing. I learned that behind every bodybuilder on stage there is a great, dedicated team. I had the very best. The encouragement of Joe, his staff, and even their families is awesome and contagious.
>
> It has been amazing to learn from Joe that many of the nutrition ideas I thought to be factual were actually misconceptions that were working against me. I'm thankful Joe has been dedicated to putting his knowledge down on paper. His nutrition manual is the only one in my home. I put it to the test. It worked. Now I'm a 65-year-old woman with a body better than some 20-year-olds. That's proof enough for me.
>
> Share your ultimate goal with Joe, have the right attitude and determination, and he'll see that you achieve it. He encourages you beyond what you think your body is capable. I have complete faith and trust in Joe.

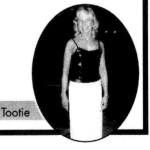

Tootie

If you're tracking this data carefully, you'll see why I stated that overall calorie intake is still always the first step. Total calorie consumption is taken care of by eating within the boundaries of your personal macronutrient range. If you're taking in a moderate amount of fat, even unsaturated fats, a great deal of it can end up stored as fat if carbs and/or overall calories are too high. (Remember the 3% rule from the last paragraph.) However, if your overall calorie intake is lower than your metabolic rate requires, you'll end up using that dietary fat as well as stored fat between meals.

So, if so much of dietary fat ends up being stored as body fat, why not just eliminate it completely? Recall that essential fatty acids play a role in hormone production as well as cellular repair, immune function, and many other life processes. If one is deficient in these essential fatty acids, health consequences cumulatively add physical stress to the body. Another key reason is the focus on keeping blood sugar moderated. Fat takes longer to digest and slows the digestion and assimilation of carbohydrates, so insulin spiking is less of a problem. This type of fat intake has merit, but only if the percentages are representative of an overall calorie intake that's low enough to cause a caloric deficit. As already discussed in detail, the relationship between fats and carbohydrates is very important. If fat intake, for example, is 25% of the total calories instead of 15%, a little lower carbohydrate intake will be necessary to accommodate the additional dietary fat. However, lowering the carbohydrates may then make the practicality of food intake difficult, and energy levels may drop. Thus, a slightly lower fat intake, allowing for more carbohydrates, may be necessary. Some flexibility between carbohydrates and fat is allowed in the Diet Docs' Rx and you shouldfeel comfortable trying different combinations as long as you stay within both ranges.

(Figure 5:3) Saturated Fat Reducing Tips

1) Use non-stick cooking spray to reduce fat or use unsaturated oils to increase "good" fat when cooking.
2) Boil, roast, bake, or steam food in place of frying.
3) Use egg whites in place of whole eggs when baking. Two egg whites equal one whole egg.
4) Use skim milk in place of whole or 2% milk.
5) Choose low- or no-fat yogurts, mayo, and salad dressings.
6) Use spices and fat-free condiments such as salsa to spice up food.
7) Use applesauce in place of butter and/or oil in baked goods.
8) Make sure canned tuna, chicken, and other meats are packed in water, not oil.
9) Choose the leanest cuts of meat.
10) Trim fat from meat.

AVERAGE JOE PHYSIOLOGY

Avoid Fat Altogether?

The question of which is worse – excess dietary fat or excess carbohydrates in relation to cardiovascular disease – is still largely misunderstood. Even if you're only 20 years old, this is a concept to understand completely. Coronary artery blockage often invokes the imagery of some fatty deposits that can be scoured away with proper eating and exercise at will. The truth is that the atherosclerotic fat that collects on the artery walls starts a process that isn't entirely reversible. The plaque that forms creates an inflammatory condition by which collagen also collects, creating a fibrous lesion. Even as plaque and cholesterol are reduced through diet and exercise, some narrowing of the vessels remain permanent. The answer is to be responsible and heart-healthy early in life and maintain it.

The average American diet includes 40% of calories from fat. Though 20 to 30% is more appropriate, that still leaves a large amount of calories that one can actively choose from unsaturated, natural sources, or from saturated and trans-fatty acids. Obviously the latter will perpetuate the process of heart disease but many choose another avenue of proactive dieting. Some are swayed to decrease overall fat consumption as low as possible and eat more carbohydrates to replace those calories. Studies show that type of dieting can lower LDL-cholesterol levels, but it also tends to lower "good" HDL-cholesterol levels and can increase triglyceride levels. When replacing carbohydrates with monounsaturated natural oils, studies show a decrease in triglycerides and an increase in HDL's. Polyunsaturated oils did decrease LDL's but didn't have much of an effect on HDL's or triglycerides. For heart health, the best combination is to keep carbohydrates low enough so that saturated fats can be replaced by some monounsaturated fats. (Olive oil and almonds are two of the richest sources of monounsaturated fats.)

A discussion of fat intake and dietary theory wouldn't be complete without commenting on the ketogenic (low-carb) camp. What do we do with the "experts" that would have us eat unlimited amounts of fat and protein but eschew carbs with the promise of a lean, muscular physique? Since excess carbs are easily converted to body fat and lead to insulin-induced lethargy, higher risk of diabetes and heart disease, and many other health perils, it's correct applied knowledge to control carbs and their quality. It's also imperative to make sure that carbs are low enough to not supply all the energy requirements of the body. A high-carb diet in which protein and fat intake is low will not allow for much body fat loss because the body will have little reason to access a secondary energy source such as body fat. If you take the opposite extreme and eliminate almost all carbohydrates from the body, then stored fat will be released at a very rapid rate. Though seemingly used successfully by many bodybuilders, this type of dieting has its problems. First, adipose cells release fat to be used as energy in the form of glycerol and fatty acids. Body cells intake the glycerol and fatty acids to metabolize them into energy through the Kreb's cycle, but glucose fragments *must* be present. (Hmm . . . looks like my physiology professor was right, fat is burned in the flames of carbohydrates.) Let me repeat this: glucose fragments (carbs) must be present to burn body fat for energy through the very efficient Kreb's cycle within every cell; but it isn't the only way. If glucose isn't available, fatty acids can combine with each other to form ketone bodies that can also be used by most cells for energy conversion. The rate of body fat usage for energy can be great using this method of diet, but the problems with this mechanism are many.

(Figure 5:4) The Dynamic Nature of Energy

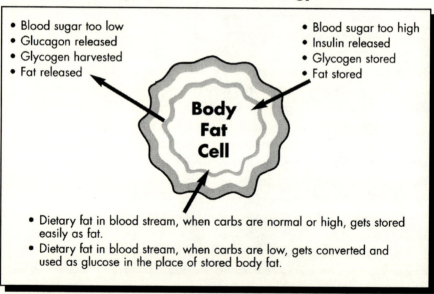

Ketogenic dieting may be effective only if fat intake isn't too excessive. Remember, adipose cells are just waiting to suck in new fat to store after meals. One of the two greatest problems of low-carb dieting is that carbs are the most protein-sparing nutrient we eat. If carbs are too low for too long, you'll lose muscle no matter how much protein you eat, period! Secondly, the brain and nervous system prefer glucose, not ketone bodies, for energy. Low energy and inefficient nervous system activity leave workouts low-key, weak, and less effective—not to mention fatigue in daily life. If you enjoy feeling lousy, having no energy, craving carbohydrates intensely, and being prone to binging, then low-carb dieting is for you. Ketogenic dieting certainly allows you to burn more fat initially because of the immense carb deficit, but increasing fat intake too much can cause a great deal of fat storage. Two steps forward, two steps back. The few who have successfully employed this type of dieting leave me wondering how much easier it would have been had they dieted "correctly" in the first place.

So, what's the take-home message about fat? If you're in a maintaining, isocaloric stage of non-dieting, you can successfully eat 30% or more of your calories from fat sources without a problem—though I would chose approximately 20% of your total so that more protein and/or carbs can be consumed. The key is in the word "isocaloric," or eating the same amount of total calories that your body uses for energy, so that whatever ratios you chose, you won't store new body fat. If you're dieting to a very low level, you can save yourself from taking too many steps backward by cutting fat intake to 10 to 15% of total calories. This simply means less fat will be available for storage after meals and the amount of stored fat used between meals for energy will be coming from a faster-shrinking supply. I wouldn't recommend staying too low for too long, though, as you may trigger the metabolic ill effects of too low a fat intake. Carbohydrate control and planning are just as important as dietary fat, but in reality the two go hand-in-hand. Many people who obsess about carbs alone end up snacking on too many nuts, extra peanut butter, and other high-fat, low-carb foods, only to increase direct fat storage from the increased fat intake. When taking in a limited amount of fat, be sure to make the most of what you get and supplement with essential fatty acids. Don't lose sight of the big picture: dietary fat intake is a critical part of your success, but it has to be just one piece of a comprehensive plan to work!

One last word about fats: have a steak once in awhile. A small percentage of saturated fat isn't going to throw you into cardiac arrest, and if your cholesterol is actually too low, you can suffer from low energy, low hormonal levels, and even depression. This is admittedly a low population, but does happen, especially with those who are very disciplined and deep into a weight-loss cycle.

CHAPTER FIVE KEY POINTS

1) Saturated fats are found primarily in animal sources.

2) Saturated fats lead to heart disease and body fat.

3) Unsaturated fats contain essential fatty acids that are necessary for many body processes.

4) Unsaturated fats in the right amounts are necessary to lose the maximal amount of body fat and to build muscle.

CHAPTER SIX

PROTEIN

So Many Choices!

Just as most saturated fats come from animal sources, so does protein. Houston, we have a problem. We need protein, but we don't want saturated fat. Fish, chicken and turkey breast, ostrich, egg whites, and even soy-based meat substitutes offer an alternative to foods high in saturated fat like beef, pork, dairy products, and whole eggs. These healthier foods are now commonly found on the menus of most restaurants making it easier to obtain on the go.

Another convenient protein choice comes in the form of protein powders, shakes, and bars. The reason professional athletes endorse supplement companies (besides getting paid) is that they actually use their products. It can be a lot easier to get supplemental protein in the form of a great tasting shake or bar, especially in on-the-run situations. We couldn't eat properly and still see a high volume of patients and clients without an occasional bar or shake to supplement our whole-food meals. Getting some of your protein from sources like shakes and bars will also help you avoid feeling like you're growing a beak from eating so much poultry!

Why Protein?

Most bodybuilders would correctly tell you that you need protein to build muscle. They would probably also tell you, however, that you need two to three times what you really require. If you asked a vegetarian about protein, you might learn how to make a dozen eggs last for a year. Your body has the ability to survive either extreme, but you will pay the price for each. You can survive without much protein at all, but you will strip the muscle right off your bones and impair your ability to build the healthiest cells.

Metabolic Transformation in Action

You've probably heard a lot of successful dieters say, "If I can lose weight on this diet, anyone can!" But in the case of Dr. Joe's plan, it really is true!

I had all the normal "excuses" for not being able to lose weight. I was over 40, had an autoimmune disorder that affected my joints, many other medical conditions, and a "sluggish" metabolism. Some doctors even suggested I just be satisfied with maintaining my current weight. But at 5'4" and 260 pounds, my blood pressure, blood sugar, and cholesterol were at life-threatening levels. I started on a diet program from a popular diet book and made some progress. It wasn't specific enough to help me when I "got stuck." I started regaining the weight without any idea how to reverse it. By June 2003 I was completely convinced that no diet would ever help me.

I called Dr. Joe, we decided to meet, and the rest is "history."

As of October 2005, I have lost over 120 pounds and am close to my goal – weighing 130 pounds after losing 130 pounds. My latest cholesterol test (non-fasting) was 178, compared to totals in the 220's before. My blood sugar is within normal levels and I hope to be free of all blood pressure medicines in the next few months. My joint problems have all but disappeared, along with my other health problems. No one recognizes the "old me" and I have no intention of going back there.

So what makes his diet and exercise plan different? For one thing, you don't start eating special foods that help you lose weight as long as you're on them – but let you regain your weight once you return to normal eating. You start by gaining an awareness of the protein, fat, and carbohydrate balances in the foods you currently eat. It was a huge wakeup call for me – mainly the carbohydrates. I had no idea I was eating so many carbs in a day. Just understanding that problem started me down the road to better eating. Dr. Joe wants you to understand the importance of looking at the foods you normally eat. I was able to look for the foods I liked, find out how to moderate them, or substitute them, and design my own plan for diet success. I put the counts of the foods I normally ate into an Excel spreadsheet. I still carried the "food count" book with me so I could calculate the values for new foods. If you can control the portions and fit the counts into your daily diet, no food is completely off limits. Joe's plan lets you take ownership of your own diet plan. With my busy schedule, I frequently ate in restaurants and have still been successful with the diet.

continued ⟶

Metabolic Transformation in Action

> He also helped me understand the importance of not only aerobic but also strength exercises and has helped guide me to an effective training program. I'm still "perfecting" that part! I am not a bodybuilder or an athletic person – I have trouble with coordination (walking and chewing gum!). I always thought my lack of skills would hamper my effectiveness with exercise. Not true.
>
> I'm still not coordinated, I'm still not a bodybuilder, but I am getting to be a thinner, fitter person thanks to this plan. I'm a normal, everyday person. Believe me, if I can do it, so can you!
>
> Does the plan work? You can probably tell from my "before" and "after" photos the answer is yes! All I can say is I used to be a size 22 and now I'm a size 4. How many 46-year-olds weigh what they did at age 18 after spending years and years well over 200 pounds? It's safe to say that reading his book and following his advice has changed my life forever. He has given me the specific tools to keep this up and to help myself recover from those inevitable "holiday" relapses!
>
> I can't thank him enough. But I can encourage all of you – it's never too late and you can do it!

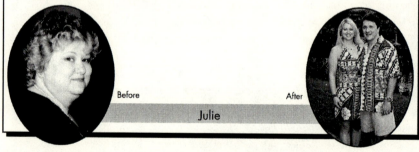
Before After
Julie

Too much protein, as advocated by some muscle magazines (owned by protein supplement companies), and you may spend a lifetime in a state of acidosis creating a host of degenerative diseases. Others warn you could end up on the kidney transplant waiting list. So, how much is best? Kind of an important question, don't you think?

The amounts of protein we advocate are designed to abundantly meet the body's requirements without the risk of undesirable effects. Protein is very important in creating new cells, such as red blood cells, skin cells, liver cells, etc., as well as in the maintenance and metabolic activities of every system in your body. If protein intake is too low, your entire body eventually suffers, even your immune system. At first, you can withstand protein depletion very efficiently because you have so much stored. Protein is broken down into amino acids, which are used in just about every chemical reaction that takes place within your body.

(Figure 6:1) **Protein Utilization**

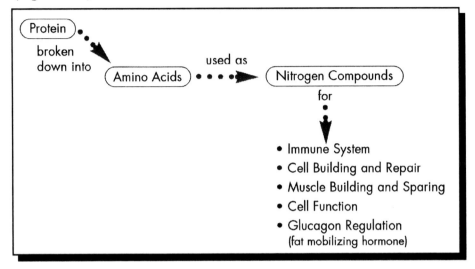

Amino acids are made up of nitrogen compounds that circulate in your bloodstream and are stored in a few places, mostly as skeletal muscle and some in the liver. So yes, you can live a long time without protein, and even longer with insufficient amounts of protein; your body will simply break down your muscle tissue to provide what it needs. It's a great survival mechanism, but as far as I'm concerned, I don't want to knowingly lose any muscle and neither should you.

We estimate protein requirements for active people. If you aren't performing rigorous exercise at least three to four times per week, choose the lower end of suggested protein ranges shown in chapter two. If you train extremely hard or perform several sessions of cardiovascular work per week, you may actually need to go slightly above the suggested amount.

Variety is the Spice of Life

Every protein has a specific amino acid profile. This means each protein source may be higher or lower in certain amino acids than other protein sources. There are many rating scales that attempt to build a hierarchy among protein sources by assigning values and deeming them "high-" or "low-quality" protein sources. There is merit to these types of ratings. However, even the highest-rated protein source is low in certain amino acids, and vice versa.

Vegetarians may have also heard that you have to combine certain foods to "make a complete protein." You're covered on this principle on two different fronts. First, digestion, absorption, and circulation keep the amino acids that you consume available for hours, and they can be augmented with other amino acids in previous or later meals. The liver also stores a small reserve of amino acids that it uses when necessary. While we're on the subject of protein and vegetarianism, I want to make sure you understand you can succeed without animal protein. I still recommend getting at least the minimal suggested protein intake in your Diet Docs' Rx for all the reasons discussed above. Think about it: if you avoid protein as a vegetarian, most of your food will come from carbohydrates causing the same physiological and behavioral challenges to health and weight loss. I have had many vegetarian clients lose weight, drop their cholesterol, and regain surprising energy by trimming starch and adding a couple protein shakes a day or other protein source acceptable to them.

The bottom line, therefore, is simply to enjoy a variety of protein sources throughout your day so that you take in a variety of amino acids. Keep in mind that saturated fats should be kept to a minimum so your diet leaves room for high-quality unsaturated fats and essential fatty acids.

Back to Hormones

Just as carbohydrates can affect your body in a positive or negative way through the modulation of the hormone insulin, protein creates a similar effect through the hormone glucagon. To oversimplify, insulin is released when you eat carbs; glucagon is released when you eat protein. Just as insulin is a storage hormone, glucagon is a retrieval, or mobilizing, hormone. It actually promotes glucose to be used as energy. When glucose isn't present in large enough quantities (because you've been so good at limiting your carbs and sticking to your daily totals!) glucagon helps mobilize body fat to be burned as energy. Hence the importance of breaking your daily macronutrient totals up so that you can have protein in most meals.

Think of insulin and glucagon as representing two opposite metabolic stimuli. Insulin is present, active, and dominant if carbohydrate intake is too high, and your body is thus in a storage mode. Glucagon is present, active, and dominant when carbohydrate intake is lower and protein intake is higher, thus promoting fat mobilization. Glucagon is one of several hormones that can "unlock" body fat cells and is the most powerful that is nutrition-dependent. Others are more exercise-dependent. When you combine the most effective nutrition and exercise to maximize these hormones, you truly are working with your body for the fastest progress.

AVERAGE JOE PHYSIOLOGY

Why Protein Helps

High-protein, low-carb diets have cycled into the diet fad rotation about every 20 years since the 1950s. Though we can all agree that carbohydrates are a critical – maybe the most important – variable in dieting, it can be taken to an unhealthy and even dangerous level. Many of these diets allow unlimited amounts of protein as long as carbs stay ultra-low. Naysayers claim that too high of a protein intake can be stressful to the kidneys, but however logical, very little evidence exists to support kidney damage. Yet there are other reasons to avoid this extreme approach.

First, studies show a very high incidence of weight regain, often with decreased lean body mass. Eliminating carbohydrates will reduce blood levels of insulin – a very good thing – but to such a low level that your body becomes very insulin sensitive. A significant hormone, adipsin, works inside the body fat cell to help regulate how much blood glucose will get pulled into the cell to be stored as fat. Its activation is modulated by insulin. Since ketogenic metabolism is less efficient than glucose metabolism, the body becomes more sensitive to glucose as it desperately wants to use it for energy. When in this hyper-sensitive state, the hormone adipsin has been measured to be many times more effective at storing glucose as body fat. This is the basis of the "starvation-mode" cliché often used as an excuse for not losing weight. The truth is, one has to be consuming virtually no carbohydrates for approximately eight weeks to have an appreciable change, but if one remains on a very-low carb diet, adipsin sensitivity will happen. The body literally becomes a fat-*storing* machine. The process will reverse itself as carbohydrate intake increases, but in the meantime, much body fat may be regained.

The second most important reason to avoid low-carb diets is the negative effect they have on mood and brain function. The brain cannot use free fatty acids for energy, has very little amounts of glycogen stores, and consumes a whopping 20% of the body's total energy at rest. It can use ketone bodies as energy in a fasting state, but mental function is greatly compromised. Eating moderate carbs is a prescription for success as well as for a sharp noodle!

Protein also has the greatest "thermic potential" among macronutrients. This means that when you eat protein, your metabolism rises because protein digestion requires more energy. Protein is very important for health and body composition, but in most cases it is deficient in the American diet. This, along with hormonal considerations such as glucagon, is the reason many new studies are showing that diets higher in protein and lower (notice we say "lower" and not "low") in carbs can cause twice as much body fat loss—even with the same amount of calories!

Scott and I often recommend that if you're "starving" and just have to have a little more food on a particular day than your macronutrient range allows, it's better to eat a little more protein than to end up binging. But if you do this too often you'll find overall calories too high and insulin will once again be a factor in keeping you from losing as much weight. Remember that calories (overall energy intake) are always step one.

CHAPTER SIX KEY POINTS

1) Protein is found in animal meats and sometimes in small amounts in certain beans and plants.

2) Supplemental protein can be found in many types of protein shakes and bars.

3) Protein is necessary for many vital processes in the body as well as muscle growth.

4) Protein sources have different amino acid profiles, making it advantageous to vary your protein choices.

5) Eating protein raises your metabolism, and through the actions of the hormone glucagon, assists you in losing body fat faster.

CHAPTER SEVEN

MEAL RATIOS

Better Living through Chemistry

Few authors have ever validated their "diets" with actual research. The reason we have been tossed to and fro, from one diet to another, is that they promise great results; but unfortunately their diets are physiologically unverified. For the average person, nutrition is often a black hole of mystery and marketing. Only recently have scientists started conducting thorough research on food's affect on health and body composition. Hormones, exercise, and food all affect nutritional status. Obviously, the fuel we put in our bodies multiple times a day is the key factor.

Measuring Cups and Calculators

Reviewing much of what we've discussed already will help to pull this section together. Eating the right amount of food per day (The Diet Docs' Rx) and dividing that food into small meals (power spacing) are the first steps in creating your eating structure. We have also established the importance of each macronutrient and some of the better choices of each. The big questions, then, are: do I have to have the same amount of protein, carbs, and fat in each meal? And, do I have to have the same ratios of nutrients in each meal?

Let me preface the following explanation with the answer, "Yes and no." To allow some flexibility, I suggest a small range in each macronutrient rather than a rigid amount of food per meal or per day. I'll explain my rationale, but first let me offer that once you are locked into a "normal" eating pattern within your daily totals, you will achieve the best results if your meals represent a fairly even distribution of macronutrients throughout the day. Consuming 60 grams of carbs in a meal and 10 in the next just isn't going to cut it. You want a good ratio of nutrients in each meal to promote stable blood sugar levels and therefore stable energy and less hunger.

Metabolic Transformation in Action

I have struggled with my weight since I was in my late 20's after I delivered our daughter, Sarah. Each year I gained a few pounds until at 49 years of age I weighed over 200. Because weight was such an issue in my family growing up, I had sworn off all diets. I didn't really eat a lot of food, but was eating all the wrong foods. But, during all those years, I continued exercising three to five times a week – walking, riding my bike, swimming, tennis, etc. So, for a heavy woman, I was in fairly good shape. Paul, as a farmer, was always very active. He, like me, was gaining a few pounds each year. His doctor told him that he needed to lose weight, especially since his cholesterol was high. In 2003, I was unable to exercise consistently at all. I was student teaching the first half of the year, and beginning a new position at the University of Southern Indiana as a math instructor the second half of the year. I was so busy that I had no time to exercise or to cook. At least two to three times week we went out to eat fast food – cheeseburgers, french fries, and Coke – food I never thought I could live without. Because I wasn't able to exercise, my weight ballooned to 218. By December 2003 I was experiencing a lot of knee pain and shoulder pain. I was also very tired and just sick of living like this. I was finally ready to change my eating habits.

We had heard about Dr. Joe and his eating plan two years prior. I e-mailed him and set up an appointment in January. I knew that if I didn't do it then, I wouldn't feel like it in January. I remember going to that first appointment thinking, "What am I doing? I am still so snowed under from my job, I can't put any effort into this now." But, I also knew that if I didn't do it now, I wouldn't do it later. Paul agreed to go with me, knowing that he needed to lose too. He didn't want to go on any diet, because he was afraid that we would just gain it back. We met with Dr. Joe and he explained the physiology of eating and losing weight. I had told myself that, yes, I needed to lose weight, but, more importantly, I needed to learn how to eat right. Dr. Joe gave us each our plan of right eating – the amount of protein, carbs, and fat we should eat each day and how to put them together. Then he sent us home to implement it. We ate our last fast food dinner and went to bed. We got up the next morning and looked at each other – where do we begin? Dr. Joe had given us a sample menu for one day, but we were totally clueless on the nutritional value of any food. The first few days (and weeks) were difficult as we were struggling to put our foods together and staying under our prescribed amount of protein, carbs, and fat. I started

continued ⟶

Metabolic Transformation in Action

> a spreadsheet to help us add up our grams each day. We soon realized that starting at dinner and planning backwards was the key for us. The eating plan allowed us the freedom to eat what we like, within reason. It didn't stop us from eating out or eating with our friends. It just gave us the tools and the information we needed to make our eating healthy, yet, fit our likes.
>
> Every Wednesday morning Paul and I would weigh in front of each other and mark our progress. We still do that to this day. The eating plan worked like clockwork. Each week I lost about one to one and a half pounds and Paul would lose one and a half to two pounds. By the end of May, Paul had lost 50 pounds, meeting his goal of 175. I continued on, losing 75 pounds by the middle of October, and meeting my goal of 145. As I began eating better, I also began training to walk/run the mini-marathon in Indianapolis. By April, I had lost 35 pounds and finished a min-marathon in less than 3 hours. By October, I was down to my goal weight and participated in my second mini-marathon in Evansville and finished in just over two and a half hours. Paul continues farming and working outside each day. We both feel so much better. My knees and shoulders don't hurt anymore. We both have more energy, and love being able to go into any store and buy clothes without trying them on. I used to wear a size 22, but now I wear a size 10. Paul went from a size 38 to a size 34. Our eating plan has become a change of life for us. We will never look on food the same. We don't always eat like we should, but we keep close tabs on our weight and adjust our eating to match. Many people have followed Dr. Joe's plan after seeing what we were able to do.

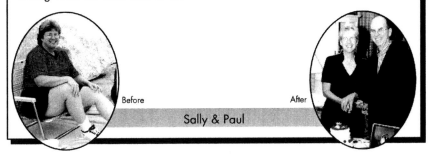

Before   After

Sally & Paul

There are, however, times when some flexibility is not only helpful, but simply the right thing to do. For example, if you've just performed an intense workout, your next meal may include a little higher percentage of carbohydrates to refill the stored glycogen (sugar) used in the muscle tissue. If you're going to bed soon, and you're

AVERAGE JOE PHYSIOLOGY

Okay, So You Can Blame Mom and Dad a Little

Though genetics are often wrongly blamed for weight management woes, it would be a great mistake to dismiss the subject. As much as we have learned about genetics in the last generation, it is a case of "the more you learn; the more you realize you don't know." Two clear issues regarding weight gain genetics are body fat cell volume and hormones that control hunger. We all have a genetic range of body fat cells that we will be born with. The proliferation of these cells is greatest during the first year of life and then a second surge is possible during puberty. It is difficult to actually increase the number of body fat cells at other times except in the case of extreme and rapid weight gain. Most fat storage is done within the number of body fat cells already created. However, this can be a wide range, for example, 15 billion in 1 person or 250 billion in another. The sheer cell mass of the extra fat cells is significant but more of a factor is that fat cells don't remain "empty." Triglycerides can be removed and kept to a minimum but the dynamic activity of metabolism makes it likely that small amounts of reserves will be left. This also increases the body's ability and ease of storing body fat – a major disadvantage. Multiply that by an exponentially large amount of body fat cells and it's easy to see how some people have "bigger frames," have "always been hefty", and have similar genetic shapes compared to parents and siblings. This isn't a life-sentence to be or remain obese, but it certainly makes it more challenging for some.

Leptin is a hormone discovered to control hunger and could be a key component in obesity and potentially a future pharmacological focus on treating it. Body fat cells secret leptin into the bloodstream proportionately to the amount of stored triglycerides. The hormone decreases hunger. This discovery gives credence to the "set point" theory describing that our bodies have a "preferred" weight. If the message isn't being transmitted properly that "there is enough fat stored," a person wouldn't feel satisfied and would continue to eat. This is a very exciting area of study but no one knows the outcome or possible side effects as of yet. Diet and exercise, though, work every time.

hungry, it would be better to have a higher percentage of protein and less carbs. This will actually stimulate more growth hormone to be released at night and suppress insulin, which inhibits growth hormone. You will also find that you're hungrier during some points of the day than you are at others. You may need a small meal only two hours after eating during the morning, but you can go three hours after lunch. Some meals will be larger, and some smaller. The point is: flexibility is often helpful due to schedules, is often physiologically necessary, and can help with your own compliance to succeed with this new eating pattern. There is a balance, however, between what is right and perfect nutritionally and the level you can achieve in your daily life.

CHAPTER SEVEN KEY POINTS

1) Keep nutrient totals spaced throughout meals.

2) Allow yourself flexibility when necessary regarding meal ratios but stay within your nutrient totals for the day.

3) Remember power spacing!

4) Learn your body's natural hunger patterns and adjust meal spacing accordingly, allowing for some flexibility.

CHAPTER EIGHT

RECIPES AND FOOD PREPARATION

Just Tell Me What to Eat!

Most new clients sit across from me in full trust, expecting body fat loss and positive health changes similar to what they have seen in the person who referred them. Occasionally, however, someone tries to help me by offering feedback on my information or methods of delivery. I have learned a great deal and invite all the criticism and feedback that clients are willing to give, but there is one common request I always refuse. A mild version of this request is a client that asks for recipes and meal plans, and then hints at wanting the inclusion of an entire daily menu. The more severe version comes from clients who beg for a written menu to follow, or simply "won't be able to succeed." "I promise, just tell me what to eat and I'll eat it! I don't care if I eat the same thing every meal, every day!"

For this client, I predict failure. This is a client who has tried everything else and has failed more as a result of lacking initiative and discipline than due to a faulty nutrition plan. Sorry to be so blunt, but keep reading—you'll see what I mean. Though it seems easier, you don't want to follow a meal-by-meal plan written by us or anyone else. Nobody knows what foods you like, what your schedule is, or what challenges may be unique to you. You have to learn to interact with food—any food—and put it into your daily plan successfully. For the sake of reference and to start you with some ideas, though, we have provided a small number of meals for you to view as examples. But, our goal is for you to create your own food intake based on the nutritional values proposed in chapter two.

When a client comes to me through a class, a consultation, or my online program, I purposely make the first step personal menu planning. My client goes home and figures out what he or she is going to eat the next day, making the best food choices, keeping nutrient totals and meal spacing as even as possible, and creating four to six meals that fall into their personal Diet Docs' Rx. Yes, it takes a food count book, a calculator, an eraser, and a lot of patience. Once you've taken this step, however, you are well on your way to success because you have a framework from which to build a pattern. You will quickly learn to substitute a variety of food and meal choices and stay within your plan. Without this planning, you will likely not be able to continue successfully. The responsibility we ask you to assume is the driving force that makes the nutritional elements work in your daily life. You will learn to adapt, be creative, and begin an ongoing process of cumulative learning. You will become your own best nutritionist. You will succeed.

Yet, many people who join a "weight-loss center" end up gaining back all the lost weight within one year. These chain weight-loss centers pride themselves on making it easy for their customers by giving them diet plans, meal cards, follow-along daily menus, and even prepackaged food. On this issue, we gladly walk in the opposite direction. Studies have determined that the majority of the people who engage in these programs weigh more one year later than the day they walked in the door. The initial ease offered by a menu is quickly complicated by the fact that you have a different schedule, different tastes, different goals, and different metabolic needs than everyone else. Secondly, you learn nothing about nutrition and how to make permanent changes unless you go through a progressive learning process. It's a little more difficult and time consuming on the front end, but the education will stick in your brain and will make it easier for the rest of your life. Your ability to control your weight will forever be greater.

What's That?

Many successful clients have suggested we write a recipe book. Maybe some day we will, but for now we have included a great recipe section for you to get started. Along with the meal samples provided, you now have a great amount of food information to help create innumerable days of good meals within your personal Rx. And, that's what it's all about: using foods you like to merge "natural" eating habits into the ranges that will accomplish your goal. Check out the book store or library for full recipe books that suit your taste and the type of meal ratios you're looking for. There are books that cater to lower-carb meals, lower-fat meals, or whatever you need help with in structuring your menu. Begin with the realization that eating the right foods in the right amounts is your focus. You don't have to make a meal for your family and a separate meal for yourself. Simply take the right foods in the right amounts. This leads to why we devalue recipes slightly. You don't have to have elaborate recipes and exotic ingredients, or even "special" foods, to diet and eat correctly. Right foods, right amounts. I can throw a can of tuna in a bowl with a cup of brown rice, stir in a half a tablespoon of flaxseed oil, pour on some salsa, and I'm ready to eat. Breakfast? No problem! Mix a scoop of strawberry protein powder into my already-cooked half-cup of oatmeal, add some almonds or oil, and I'm off to the office. Creativity! You may get some funny looks once in awhile, but you'll have the last laugh. I'm sure Scott got some snickers as he chomped on his ostrich jerky once in awhile, but he's the one who lost 60 pounds! When you put this book down tonight, take a tour of your kitchen and start looking at the three macronutrient categories on the food labels. Some will pleasantly surprise you, and some will spur you to put green Poison Control Center stickers on the box. Now you're taking an active role in your own nutrition.

Breakfast without Sugar

Most breakfast selections are a disastrous way to start your day. Sugar and refined (high-glycemic) flour are used to create very tasty cereals, as long as you don't mind a little extra body fat, low energy, and hunger. You're not a cereal person? How about a doughnut or a "healthier" refined-flour bagel with 50 grams of carbs? Breakfast bars, pastries—yep, same story.

Breakfast is actually a difficult meal for most people due to time constraints and/or a lack of food ideas. Unless you want my tuna and salsa concoction for breakfast, pay attention. Protein in the morning is difficult unless you plan ahead. Take time to cook egg white combinations or utilize a protein substitute. Scrambled egg whites (with one whole egg—if you like—and the extra fat fits in your meal plan) cooked in olive or canola oil, joined by oat or rye toast, make a great breakfast. You can even get fancy with different omelets.

Oatmeal (watch for added sugar in flavored brands) is an excellent choice and can be fortified with fat and protein, as noted earlier. Meal replacement shakes can also be very helpful. These are protein powders packaged in individual servings (or large canisters) and these products make great shakes in a blender where you can add your choice of high-quality oil and low-glycemic fruit if you chose to "spend" that amount of carbohydrate at breakfast. You can't get much quicker than that.

A thought that may help you decrease your reliance on huge amounts of processed carbs at breakfast is to view it as just another meal. Bodybuilders will sometimes eat yet another chicken breast and green beans for breakfast (gross!). You don't need to go to that extreme, but who said that we need eight ounces of juice and a stack of pancakes for breakfast? It is an important meal to not skip, but I challenge you to try increasing the protein and decreasing the carbs. You'll be less hungry in the later morning, and you'll have more energy. Plus, you will have saved more carbs for later meals and snacks. It's all good!

Lunch and Supper the Easy Way

Lunch and supper, or even whole food snacks, can easily be pieced together by combining compatible protein, carbohydrate, and fat choices. Choose your protein source and then add complimentary carbs and fat. If it's a chicken breast, decide whether you want pasta, brown rice, a sweet potato—it's your choice. Add a limited amount of a healthy fat source (if necessary to reach your suggested nutrient totals) and eat with confidence. A deli (chicken or turkey breast) sandwich can be made with low-glycemic bread and condiments. Health food stores even have mayonnaise made with canola oil instead of saturated fat. A chicken breast salad with a little Italian dressing is a great choice. The salad vegetables give you great carbs and the dressing gives you olive oil. Your creativity and planning are the only factors that can inhibit you from enjoying great tasting food and easy-to-prepare meals.

(Figure 8:1) Simple Breakfasts

Food Source	Protein	Carbs	Fat
3 egg whites	12	0	0
1 piece whole grain toast	2	13	1
1 tsp. canola oil (to cook eggs)	0	0	4
Total	14	13	5
(Great light breakfast that is very balanced and filling.)			
6 egg whites/1 yolk	27	0	6
2 pieces whole grain toast	4	26	2
1 tsp. canola oil	0	0	4
Total	31	26	12
(Similar breakfast but larger.)			
1/2 cup (dry) oats	5	27	3
1 scoop protein powder	30	5	1
1/2 tbsp. flaxseed oil	0	0	6
Total	35	32	10
Mix powder and oil into oats after oats are cooked.			
(Protein powder is optional but does significantly fortify this already great breakfast.)			
1/2 cup low-fat cottage cheese	13	4	5
4 egg whites	16	0	0
1 tsp. canola oil (to cook)	0	0	4
Chopped omelet veggies	0	3	0
Total	29	7	9
Mix cottage cheese and egg whites in bowl, then make omelet.			
(High-protein, low-carb breakfast that is versatile and tastes great.			
Add carb sources such as toast if desired.)			

Food Source	Protein	Carbs	Fat
1/2 cup low-fat, plain yogurt	8	10	2
1 scoop protein powder	30	5	1
1/8 cup almonds	3	3	7
1/4 cup (dry) oats	3	13	1
Totals	44	31	11

Mix everything together into yogurt. May substitute high-fiber cereal for oats.
May add fruit for more carbs if needed.
Cut in half if necessary for your meal plan.
(This quick option tastes like dessert for breakfast!)

Meal replacement shake	40	20	1
1/2 tbsp. flaxseed oil	0	0	5
8 oz. skim milk	8	4	2
Totals	48	24	8

May substitute 1 tbsp. peanut butter for flaxseed oil. May use water instead of milk.
Blend in mixer with ice. May use scoop of protein powder instead of meal
replacement packet to decrease protein and carbs.
(This is a quick but significant jump-start for the day.)

1 cup high-fiber cereal	3	35	1
1 cup skim milk	8	4	2
1/2 scoop protein powder	15	2	1
Totals	26	41	4

Mix vanilla protein powder well in milk, pour on cereal.
(Can't get much faster than this, but measure well; the carbs in cereal add up fast!)

3 egg whites	12	0	0
2 pieces low-fat turkey bacon	6	0	2
1 tsp. canola oil (to cook)	0	0	4
2 pieces whole grain toast	4	26	2
Totals	22	26	8

May use whole grain pancakes instead of toast. May drop 1 piece of toast to
decrease carbs. May make into sandwich.
(If you have time, this is a classic!)

(Figure 8:2) Lunch and Dinner

Food Source	Protein	Carbs	Fat
5 oz. chicken breast	35	0	5
1/2 cup rice	2	22	0
Salad or can of green beans	0	10	0
2 tbsp. low-/no-fat dressing	0	2	2
Totals	37	34	7

(This is a "full-size" lunch or supper that is complete in all categories.)

Food Source	Protein	Carbs	Fat
4 oz. deli turkey breast	28	0	4
2 pieces whole grain bread	4	26	2
Lettuce/tomato	0	0	0
Mustard	0	0	0
Totals	32	26	6

May use 1 piece of bread to decrease carbs and add a small salad to increase fiber. (A "plain 'ole sandwich" can be a great meal.)

Food Source	Protein	Carbs	Fat
4 oz. tuna	30	0	0
1 tbsp. light mayo	0	2	3
Small salad (varies)	0	10	0
5 small whole wheat crackers	0	10	2
Totals	30	22	5

(Quick and easy tuna salad.)

Food Source	Protein	Carbs	Fat
3 oz. chicken breast strips	21	0	3
1 tortilla wrap (varies)	0	5	1
Lettuce, veggie condiments	0	5	0
3-4 tbsp. salsa (varies)	0	5	0
Totals	21	15	4

(Creative and delicious!)

Food Source	Protein	Carbs	Fat
Chicken breast sandwich/sub	30	35	5

Estimate well or look up in a food count book.
Ask for no mayo, no cheese.
(Everyone's on the go sometimes!)

Food Source	Protein	Carbs	Fat
Meal replacement shake mixed in water	40	20	1
(Not the preferable whole food lunch, but quick in a pinch.)			
Protein bar (varies)	30	30	7
(Best used as a snack so you can get fiber and whole food meals, but in an emergency...)			
Small salad (varies)	0	10	0
1/2 cup low-fat cottage cheese	13	4	5
Pop-top can of chicken	13	0	1
Totals	26	14	6
(Just a quick, small lunch option.)			
4 oz. baked fish	24	0	1
1 cup steamed broccoli	0	8	0
4 oz. baked potato	1	30	0
1 tsp. butter	0	0	5
Totals	25	38	6
(A great pattern for dinner.)			
1/2 oz. almonds	3	3	6
3 oz. chicken	21	0	3
1 tbsp. light mayo	0	2	3
Dash of curry (spice)	0	0	0
2 pieces whole wheat bread	6	24	0
Totals	30	29	12
(Any recipe can be used as long as the amounts of foods used are measured and tracked. Be creative!!)			

Snacks

Snacks are vital to your plan. They keep your blood chemistry stable (as long as your food choices are appropriate), lessen hunger, help to keep you from overeating at meals, and keep your metabolism high. Convenience, however, can compromise quality if you're not careful. To keep food quality high, snacks may be an area where you need to be more flexible with the spacing of your nutrients. For example, an apple and an eighth of a cup of almonds would make a great snack of low-glycemic carbs and quality fat, but the protein is low. Making sure your protein was adequate at your previous and your next meal would therefore be imperative. There are also a few high-quality snack bars that have a balanced amount of protein, carbs, and fat. They are especially good when you crave chocolate or a treat since there are many great flavors out there. Bars come in many sizes so stick to the right amount for your meal or snack even if you have to just eat half and save the rest for later.

After-dinner snacks can consist of a small amount of carbs or a protein shake. (Keep your eyes on those serving sizes. A bag of popcorn is three servings!) Try to keep under 150 to 200 calories per late-night snack. Weight loss will be accelerated if after-dinner snacking is eliminated or minimized, so be vigilant if you find yourself snacking too heavily at night. If you eat a protein-only snack at night, you'll decrease sleeping levels of insulin and your body will release more growth hormone at night, which increases recovery from exercise and also speeds fat loss. I'll often have a scoop of protein powder, and with some creativity it becomes like dessert. For example, after I write this paragraph, as it's 10:30 at night, I'm going straight to the kitchen, mixing a scoop of banana-flavored protein powder with a tiny amount of water in a bowl, whipping it with a fork into a cake frosting consistency, crumbling in half of a graham cracker, and it tastes just like vanilla wafer banana pudding dessert. See, creativity does pay off!

(Figure 8:3) Snacks on the Run

Food Source	Protein	Carbs	Fat
Meal replacement shake mixed in water	40	20	1
Protein bar (varies)	30	30	7
1 scoop protein powder	30	5	0
1/2 C skim milk	4	5	0
1/2 C pineapple	0	15	0
1 C strawberries	1	11	0
1 tsp. flaxseed oil	0	0	4
Totals	35	36	5
(Add ice, blend, freeze, and thaw out about one hour before eating. Tastes like frozen yogurt. Or, just blend and drink!)			
1/2 C skim milk	4	5	0
1/2 scoop protein powder	15	2	0
1 tbsp. peanut butter	5	4	8
Totals	24	11	8
(You can make an infinite variety of protein shakes!)			
"Energy/snack" bar	16	24	8
Apple	1	30	0
(Yep, just an apple can be fine. Watch out though, as a stand-alone carb source you may get hungry soon after.)			
Yogurt (per label)	10	20	3

(Figure 8:4) Surviving Restaurants

1) Specify how you want food prepared to avoid added butter, etc.
2) Order baked, grilled, or broiled entrees.
3) Ask for salad dressings on the side (fat-free if possible).
4) Share a meal.
5) Ask for grilled or steamed veggies instead of potato or rice if reducing carbohydrates.
6) Use red sauces instead of cream sauces.
7) Ask for cheese, croutons, bacon, egg yolks, and nuts to be left off salad.
8) Dip fork in dressing instead of pouring dressing on salad.
9) Ask for complimentary bread or chips to not be brought to the table.
10) Use a food count book to plan and estimate food intake.
11) Ask for a nutrition facts card/menu or go to the website of your favorite restaurants so you have accurate information for your log book. That way you'll never be caught off guard.

RECIPES

DINNERS

Southwest Chicken

4 boneless skinless chicken breast halves (1 pound)
16 ounces picante sauce
2 tablespoons brown sugar
1 tablespoon mustard

Place chicken in a greased shallow 2-qt. baking dish. In a small bowl, combine the picante sauce, brown sugar, and mustard; pour over chicken. Bake, uncovered, at 400 degrees for 30-35 minutes. Serve over rice if desired.

Yield: 4 servings
Nutritional Analysis: One serving (calculated without rice) equals 224 calories, 4 g fat, 19 g carbohydrate, 28 g protein
Diabetic Exchanges: 3 lean meat, ½ starch

Light Turkey Salad Tortillas

12 ounces cooked turkey, shredded or cubed
1 cup (4 ounces) fat-free shredded cheddar cheese
¾ cup finely chopped celery
½ cup finely chopped onion
1 can (2 ¼ ounces) sliced olives, drained
½ cup light mayonnaise
¼ cup picante sauce
6 low-carb flour tortillas (7 inches)

In a bowl, combine the first 7 ingredients, mix well. Evenly divide filling on center on each tortilla. Fold sides and ends over filling, then roll up. Place in a shallow, microwave-safe dish. Cover and microwave on high for 2-3 minutes or until cheese is melted and filling is hot.

Yield: 6 servings
Nutritional Analysis: One serving equals 151 calories, 3 g fat, 16 g carbohydrate, 15 g protein
Diabetic Exchanges: ½ starch, 1 ½ meat, 1 vegetable

Lean Swedish Meatballs

2 egg whites, lightly beaten
¼ cup ketchup
¾ cup dry bread crumbs
2 tablespoons dried parsley flakes
2 tablespoons Worcestershire sauce
1 teaspoon onion powder
1 teaspoon garlic powder
1 teaspoon pepper
½ teaspoon salt
½ teaspoon chili powder
3 pounds ground turkey breast
ADDITIONAL INGREDIENTS:
2 envelopes brown gravy mix
½ cup fat-free sour cream

In a bowl, combine the first 10 ingredients. Crumble meat over mixture and mix well. Shape into 1-in. balls (about 6 dozen). Place in a single layer in ungreased 15-in. x 10-in. x 1-in. baking pans. Bake at 400 degrees for 20 minutes or until no longer pink, turning often. Remove from the oven; stir in sour cream. Cool.

Yield: 75 meatballs per batch, 15 servings
Nutritional Analysis: Five Swedish meatballs equal 223 calories, 7 g fat, 8 g carbohydrate, 32 g protein
Diabetic Exchanges: 4 lean meat, ½ starch

Blueberry Chicken

4 boneless skinless chicken breast halves (1 pound)
1 tablespoon canola oil
¼ cup apricot preserves *or* fruit spread
3 tablespoons Dijon mustard
¼ cup white wine vinegar *or* cider vinegar
1 cup fresh *or* frozen blueberries

In a large skillet over medium heat, cook chicken in oil for about 5 minutes on each side or until lightly browned. Combine preserves and mustard; spoon over chicken. Reduce heat to low; cover and simmer for 20 minutes or until chicken juices run clear.

With a slotted spoon, remove chicken and keep warm. Add vinegar to skillet; bring to a boil. Reduce heat, simmer uncovered for 3 minutes or until sauce is reduced by one-third, stirring occasionally. Stir in blueberries. Serve rice if desired.

Yield: 4 servings
Nutritional Analysis: One serving (prepared with 100% apricot fruit spread) equals 206 calories, 6 g fat, 10 g carbohydrate, 28 g protein
Diabetic Exchanges: 3 lean meat, 1 1/2 fruit

Creamy Chicken Enchiladas

1 small onion, chopped
1 can (10 ¾ ounces) reduced-fat, reduced-sodium condensed cream of chicken soup, undiluted
1 can (10 ounces) diced tomatoes and green chilies, undrained
1 cup (8 ounces) fat-free sour cream
1 cup (4 ounces) shredded fat-free cheddar cheese
1 cup (4 ounces) shredded reduced-fat mozzarella cheese
6 low-carb flour tortillas
3 cooked chicken breasts (cubed)

In a skillet or saucepan coated with nonstick cooking spray, sauté onion until tender. Remove from heat. Add soup, tomatoes, sour cream, ¾ cup cheddar cheese, and ¾ cup mozzarella cheese; mix well. Divide evenly on each tortilla, top with ½ of a cubed chicken breast. Roll up tightly.

Place seam side down in a 13-in. x 9-in. x 2-in. baking dish coated with nonstick cooking spray. Top with remaining soup mixture; sprinkle with remaining cheeses. Bake, uncovered, at 350 degrees for 20-25 minutes or until heated through.

Yield: 6 servings
Nutritional Analysis: One serving equals 226 calories, 6 g fat, 21 g carbohydrate, 22 g protein
Diabetic Exchanges: 2 lean meat, 1 ½ starch, 1 vegetable

Dill Salmon

1 salmon fillet (1 pound)
1 ½ teaspoons dill weed

½ cup fat-free plain yogurt
½ teaspoon brown sugar
½ teaspoon salt-free seasoning blend

Place the salmon in a 13-in. x 9-in. x 2-in. baking dish coated with nonstick cooking spray and sprinkle with ½ teaspoon dill. Cover and bake at 375 degrees for 20-25 minutes or until the fish flakes easily with a fork. In a small saucepan, combine the yogurt, sugar, seasoning blend, and remaining dill. Cook and stir over low heat until heated through.

Yield: 4 servings
Nutritional Analysis: One serving equals 227 calories, 12 g fat, 3 g carbohydrate, 24 g protein
Diabetic Exchanges: 2 ½ lean meat, 2 fat.

Lean and Meaty Spaghetti Sauce

1 ½ pounds ground turkey breast
½ pound bulk Italian sausage
1 medium green pepper, chopped
1 medium onion, chopped
8 garlic cloves, minced
3 cans (14 1/2 ounces *each*) diced tomatoes, drained
2 cans (15 ounces *each*) tomato sauce
2 cans (6 ounces *each*) tomato paste
¼ cup sugar
2 tablespoons Italian seasoning
1 tablespoon dried basil
1 teaspoon salt
½ teaspoon pepper
Hot cooked spaghetti

In a large skillet over medium heat, cook turkey and sausage until no longer pink; drain. Transfer to a 5-qt. slower cooker. Stir in green pepper, onion, garlic, tomatoes, tomato sauce, paste, sugar, and seasonings; mix well. Cover and cook on low for 8 hours or until bubbly. Serve over spaghetti.

Yield: 12 servings
Nutritional Analysis: One serving (calculated without spaghetti—add macronutrient values for amount of spaghetti served) equals 180 calories, 4 g fat, 12 g carbohydrate, 24 g protein

Diabetic Exchanges: 1 starch, 2 meat, 1 vegetable

Italian Orange Roughy Fillets

1 pound orange roughy fillets
½ cup tomato juice
1 tablespoon white vinegar
1 envelope Italian salad dressing mix
¼ cup chopped green onions
¼ cup chopped green pepper

Place fish fillets in a shallow 2-qt glass baking dish, positioning the thickest portion of fish toward the outside edges. Combine tomato juice, vinegar, and salad dressing mix; pour over fish. Cover and refrigerate for 30 minutes.

Sprinkle with onions and green pepper. Cover and bake at 400 for 15 minutes or until fish flakes easily with a fork. Let stand, covered, for 2 minutes.

Yield: 4 servings
Nutritional Analysis: One serving equals 122 calories, 2 g fat, 5 g carbohydrate, 21 g protein
Diabetic Exchanges: 2 very lean meat

Oriental Sesame Chicken

1 pound boneless skinless chicken breasts, cubed
1 tablespoon canola oil
¼ cup light soy sauce
¼ cup sesame seeds
1 large onion, sliced
2 jars (4 1/2 ounces *each*) sliced mushrooms, drained, *or* 2 cups sliced fresh mushrooms

In a large skillet, cook chicken in oil until no longer pink. Stir in the soy sauce and sesame seeds. Cook and stir over medium heat for 5 minutes. Remove chicken with a slotted spoon; set aside and keep warm. In the same skillet, sauté onion and mushrooms until onion is tender. Return chicken to pan; heat through.

Yield: 4 servings

Nutritional Analysis: One serving equals 212 calories, 8 g fat, 6 g carbohydrate, 29 g protein
Diabetic Exchange: 4 very lean meat, 1 fat, 1 vegetable

Light Spinach Quiche

3 ounces fat-free cream cheese
1 cup skim milk
8 egg whites
¼ teaspoon pepper
3 cups (12 ounces) shredded fat-free cheddar cheese
1 package (10 ounces) frozen chopped spinach, thawed and squeezed dry
1 cup frozen chopped broccoli, thawed and well-drained
1 small onion, finely chopped
5 fresh mushrooms, sliced

In a small mixing bowl, beat cream cheese. Add milk, egg whites, and pepper; beat until smooth. Stir in remaining ingredients. Transfer to a 10-in quiche pan coated with nonstick cooking spray. Bake at 350 degrees for 45-50 minutes or until a knife inserted near the center comes out clean.

Yield: 8 servings
Nutritional Analysis: One serving equals 122 calories, 2 g fat, 8 g carbohydrate, 18 g protein
Diabetic Exchanges: 1 starch, 1 meat

Italian Chicken Cutlets

6 boneless skinless chicken breast halves (1 ½ pounds)
1 cup dry bread crumbs
½ cup nonfat Parmesan cheese topping
2 tablespoons wheat germ
1 teaspoon dried basil
½ teaspoon garlic powder
1 cup plain fat-free yogurt
Refrigerated butter-flavored spray

Flatten chicken to ½-in. thickness. In a shallow dish, combine the bread crumbs, Parmesan topping, wheat germ, basil, and garlic powder. Place the yogurt in another shallow dish. Dip chicken in yogurt, then coat with the crumb mixture.

Place in a 15-in. x 10-in. x 1-in. baking pan coated with nonstick cooking spray. Spritz chicken with butter-flavored spray. Bake, uncovered, at 350 degrees for 20-25 minutes or until the juices run clear.

Yield: 6 servings
Nutritional Analysis: One serving equals 270 calories, 5 g fat, 15 g carbohydrate, 32 g protein
Diabetic Exchanges: 3 lean meat, 1 starch

Chicken Veggie Stew

2 pounds boneless skinless chicken breasts, cubed
1 can (14 ½ ounces) Italian diced tomatoes, undrained
2 medium potatoes, peeled and cut into ½ inch cubes
6 medium carrots, chopped
4 celery stalks, chopped
1 large onion, chopped
1 medium green pepper, chopped
2 cans (4 ounces *each*) mushrooms, drained
2 low-sodium chicken bouillon cubes
1 teaspoon chili powder
¼ teaspoon pepper
1 tablespoon cornstarch
2 cups water

In a slow cooker, combine the first 11 ingredients. In a small bowl, combine cornstarch and water until smooth. Stir into chicken mixture. Cover and cook on low for 8-10 hours or until vegetables are tender.

Yield: 8 servings
Nutritional Analysis: One serving equals 220 calories, 4 g fat, 16 g carbohydrate, 30 g protein
Diabetic Exchanges: 2 vegetable, 3 lean meat, ½ starch

Spicy White Chili

2 pounds boneless skinless chicken breasts, cubed
1 small onion, chopped
2 cups low-sodium chicken broth
1 can (4 ounces) chopped green chilies

½ teaspoon garlic powder
½ teaspoon dried oregano
½ teaspoon minced fresh cilantro *or* parsley
¼ teaspoon cayenne pepper
1 can (15 ounces) white kidney or cannellini beans, rinsed and drained

In a saucepan coated with nonstick cooking spray, sauté chicken and onion until juices run clear; drain if desired. Stir in broth, chilies, garlic powder, oregano, cilantro, and cayenne. Bring to a boil. Reduce heat; simmer, uncovered, for 30 minutes. Stir in beans; cook 10 minutes longer.

Yield: 8 servings
Nutritional Analysis: One serving equals 220 calories, 4 g fat, 14 g carbohydrate, 32 g protein
Diabetic Exchanges: 3 ½ lean meat, 1 starch, 1 vegetable

Zesty Cod

1 ½ cups water
1 tablespoon lemon juice
2 pounds cod fillets
¼ tsp pepper
1 small onion, finely chopped
2 large tomatoes, sliced
½ cup chopped green pepper
½ cup seasoned bread crumbs
¼ cup grated, reduced-fat Parmesan cheese
½ teaspoon dried basil
1 tablespoon olive oil

In a bowl, combine the water and lemon juice. Add fish; let sit for 5 minutes. Drain and place in an 11-in. x 7-in. x 2-in. baking dish coated with nonstick cooking spray. Sprinkle with pepper. Layer with onion, tomatoes, and green pepper. Combine the remaining ingredients, sprinkle over top. Bake, uncovered, at 375 degrees for 20-30 minutes or until fish flakes easily with a fork.

Yield: 8 servings
Nutritional Analysis: One serving equals 188 calories, 4 g fat, 10 g carbohydrate, 28 g protein
Diabetic Exchanges: 3 lean meat, 1 starch

Creamed Mushroom Turkey

1 boneless turkey breast (3 pounds), halved
1 tablespoon canola oil-based butter, melted
2 tablespoons dried parsley flakes
½ teaspoon dried tarragon
½ teaspoon salt
¼ teaspoon pepper
1 jar (4 ½ ounces) sliced mushrooms, drained *or* 1 cup sliced fresh mushrooms
½ cup chicken broth
2 tablespoons cornstarch
¼ cup cold water

Place the turkey in a slow cooker. Brush with butter. Sprinkle with parsley, tarragon, salt, and pepper. Top with mushrooms. Pour broth over all. Cover and cook on low for 7-8 hours. Remove turkey and keep warm. Skim fat from cooking juices. In a saucepan, combine cornstarch and water until smooth. Gradually add cooking juices. Bring to a boil; cook and stir for 2 minutes or until thickened. Serve over the turkey.

Yield: 12 servings
Nutritional Analysis: One serving equals 191 calories, 7 g fat, 4 g carbohydrate, 28 g protein
Diabetic Exchanges: 3 lean meat, ½ vegetable

Curry Chicken Breasts

4 boneless skinless chicken breast halves (4 ounces each)
1 tablespoon canola oil
¼ cup Worcestershire sauce
2 tablespoons chili sauce
2 teaspoons curry powder
1 teaspoon garlic powder
¼ teaspoon hot pepper sauce
¼ cup chopped onion

In a large skillet, brown chicken on both sides in oil. In a bowl, combine the Worcestershire sauce, chili sauce, curry powder, garlic powder, and hot pepper sauce. Pour over chicken. Add onion. Reduce heat; cover and simmer for 9-11 minutes.

Yield: 4 servings

Nutritional Analysis: One serving equals 186 calories, 6 g fat, 4 g carbohydrate, 28 g protein
Diabetic Exchanges: 3 lean meat, 1 vegetable

Parmesan Chicken

½ cup dry bread crumbs
½ cup grated reduced-fat Parmesan cheese
2 tablespoons minced fresh parsley
1 garlic clove, minced
¼ teaspoon pepper
4 egg whites
8 boneless skinless chicken breast halves (2 pounds)
½ cup sliced almonds
Butter-flavored cooking spray

In a shallow bowl, combine the first 5 ingredients. In another shallow bowl, beat the egg whites. Dip chicken in egg whites, then coat with crumb mixture. Place in a 13-in. x 9-in. x 2-in. baking dish coated with nonstick cooking spray. Sprinkle almonds over chicken. Spritz lightly with butter-flavored spray. Bake, uncovered, at 350 degrees for 30 minutes.

Yield: 8 servings
Nutritional Analysis: One serving equals 216 calories, 8 g fat, 6 g carbohydrate, 30 g protein
Diabetic Exchanges: 3 lean meat, ½ starch

Mini Turkey Loaves

4 egg whites
½ cup fat-free plain yogurt
1 can (6 ounces) tomato paste
2 tablespoons Worcestershire sauce
½ cup quick-cooking oats
1 small onion, chopped
2 tablespoons dried parsley flakes
1 teaspoon salt
½ teaspoon garlic powder
½ teaspoon pepper

2 pounds ground turkey breast
½ cup low-carb ketchup

In a large bowl, combine the first 10 ingredients. Crumble turkey over mixture and mix well. Shape into eight loaves. Place on a rack coated with nonstick cooking spray in a shallow baking pan. Bake, uncovered, at 350 degrees for 30 minutes. Spoon ketchup over the loaves. Bake 15 minutes longer.

Yield: 8 servings
Nutritional Analysis: One serving equals 172 calories, 4 g fat, 2 g carbohydrates, 30 g protein
Diabetic Exchanges: 3 lean meat, 1 starch, ½ fat

Sweet and Spicy Chicken

1 pound boneless skinless chicken breasts, cut into ½ inch cubes
3 tablespoons taco seasoning
1 tablespoon canola oil
1 jar (11 ounces) chunky salsa
½ cup sugar-free peach preserves

Coat chicken with taco seasoning. In a skillet, brown chicken in oil. Combine salsa and preserves; stir into skillet. Bring to a boil. Reduce heat; cover and simmer for 2-3 minutes. Serve over rice if desired.

Yield: 4 servings
Nutritional Analysis: One serving equals 197 calories, 5 g fat, 10 g carbohydrate, 28 g protein
Diabetic Exchanges: 3 lean meat, 1 fruit, ½ fat

Lemon Baked Salmon

1 salmon fillet (2 pounds)
2 tablespoons canola oil-based butter
¼ cup white wine
2 tablespoons lemon juice
½ teaspoon pepper
½ teaspoon dried tarragon
Sliced lemon

Pat salmon dry. Place in a greased 13-in. x 9-in. x 2-in. baking dish. Brush with butter. Combine remaining ingredients; pour over salmon. Top salmon with lemon slices. Bake, uncovered, at 425 degrees for 20-25 minutes or until fish flakes easily with a fork.

Yield: 8 servings
Nutritional Analysis: One (4-ounce) serving equals 192 calories, 8 g fat, 2 g carbohydrate, 28 g protein
Diabetic Exchanges: 4 lean meat, 1 fat

Orange Roughy Primavera

1 tablespoon canola oil-based butter
4 orange roughy fillets (4 ounces each), thawed
2 tablespoons lemon juice
Pinch pepper
1 garlic clove, minced
1 tablespoon olive oil
1 cup broccoli florets
1 cup cauliflowerets
1 cup julienned carrots
1 cup sliced fresh mushrooms
½ cup sliced celery
¼ teaspoon dried basil
¼ teaspoon salt
¼ cup reduced-fat, grated Parmesan cheese

Place butter in a 13-in. x 9-in. x 2-in. baking dish; add fish and turn to coat. Sprinkle with lemon juice and pepper. Bake, uncovered, at 450 degrees for 5 minutes. Meanwhile, in a large skillet over medium heat, sauté garlic in oil. Add the next 7 ingredients, stir-fry until vegetables are crisp-tender, about 2-3 minutes. Spoon over the fish; sprinkle with cheese. Bake, uncovered, at 450 degrees for 3-5 minutes or until fish flakes easily with a fork.

Yield: 4 servings
Nutritional Analysis: One serving equals 215 calories, 7 g fat, 10 g carbohydrate, 28 g protein
Diabetic Exchanges: 3 very lean meat, 1 ½ vegetable, 1 fat

Spicy Haddock

2 pounds haddock fillets, thawed
1 can (4 ounces) chopped green chilies
1 tablespoon canola oil
1 tablespoon soy sauce
2 tablespoons Worcestershire sauce
1 teaspoon paprika
½ teaspoon garlic powder
½ teaspoon chili powder
Dash hot pepper sauce

Place fillets in a 13-in. x 9-in. x 2-in. baking dish that has been coated with nonstick cooking spray. Combine remaining ingredients; spoon over fish. Bake, uncovered, at 350 degrees for 20-25 minutes or until fish flakes easily with a fork.

Yield: 8 servings
Nutritional Analysis: One (4-ounce) serving equals 155 calories, 5 g fat, 2 g carbohydrate, 28 g protein
Diabetic Exchanges: 3 very lean meat, ½ vegetable

Lemon Fish

1 pound whitefish *or* sole fillets
¼ cup lemon juice
1 teaspoon olive oil
2 teaspoons salt-free lemon-pepper seasoning
1 small onion, thinly sliced
1 teaspoon dried parsley flakes

Cut fish into serving-size pieces. Place in an ungreased 11-in. x 7-in. x 2-in. baking dish. Drizzle with lemon juice and oil; sprinkle with lemon pepper. Arrange onion over fish; sprinkle with parsley. Cover and let stand for 5 minutes. Bake at 350 degrees for 20 minutes or until fish flakes easily with a fork.

Yield: 4 servings
Nutritional Analysis: One serving equals 156 calories, 6 g fat, 2 g carbohydrate, 28 g protein
Diabetic Exchanges: 3 very lean meat

Turkey Tortilla Pie

1 small onion, finely chopped
½ teaspoon garlic powder
1 teaspoon olive oil
1 pound ground turkey breast
2 teaspoons chili powder
1 teaspoon dried oregano
½ teaspoon ground cumin
½ teaspoon cayenne pepper
1 can (15 ounces) black beans, rinsed and drained
1 jar (16 ounces) salsa
¾ cup low-sodium chicken broth
8 low-carb, fat-free flour tortillas
½ cup shredded reduced-fat Monterey Jack cheese
¼ cup light sour cream

In a skillet, sauté onion and garlic powder in oil until the onion is tender. Add turkey, chili powder, oregano, cumin, and cayenne, cook and stir over medium heat until turkey is no longer pink. Stir in beans. Remove from heat. Combine salsa and broth; spread a thin layer in a 2 ½-qt. baking dish coated with nonstick cooking spray. Cut tortillas into 1 inch strips and then into thirds; arrange half over salsa mixture. Top with half of the turkey mixture and half of the remaining salsa mixture. Repeat layers. Sprinkle with cheese. Cover and bake at 350 degrees for 25 minutes or until bubbly. Top servings with sour cream.

Yield: 8 servings
Nutritional Analysis: One (1 cup) serving equals 270 calories, 6 g fat, 32 g carbohydrate, 22 g protein
Diabetic Exchanges: 2 starch, 2 lean meat, 1 vegetable

Italian-Tomato Chicken

4 boneless skinless chicken breast halves (1 pound)
½ cup fat-free Italian salad dressing
8 tomato slices, ¼ inch thick
4 teaspoons seasoned bread crumbs
1 teaspoon minced fresh basil *or* ¼ teaspoon dried basil
1 tablespoon grated, reduced-fat Parmesan cheese

Place chicken in a shallow bowl; pour ¼ cup dressing over chicken. Cover and refrigerate for 2 hours. Transfer chicken to a shallow baking dish; discard marinade. Drizzle with remaining dressing. Cover and bake at 400 degrees for 10 minutes. Top each chicken breast with tomato slices, crumbs, basil, and cheese. Cover and bake for 10 minutes. Uncover and bake 10-15 minutes longer or until chicken juices run clear.

Yield: 4 servings
Nutritional Analysis: One serving equals 164 calories, 4 g fat, 8 g carbohydrate, 28 g protein
Diabetic Exchanges: 3 lean meat, ½ starch

Creamy Pea Salad

2 medium carrots, chopped
1 package (16 ounces) frozen peas
1 celery rib, thinly sliced
¼ cup cubed reduced-fat mozzarella cheese
2 green onions, thinly sliced
2 tablespoons buttermilk
2 tablespoons plain nonfat yogurt
1 teaspoon fat-free mayonnaise
½ teaspoon cider *or* red wine vinegar
½ teaspoon dried basil
¼ teaspoon pepper

In a saucepan, cook carrots in a small amount of boiling water for 2 minutes. Add peas; cook 5 minutes longer. Drain; rinse in cold water and drain again. Place in a bowl; add celery, cheese, and onions. Combine remaining ingredients; pour over pea mixture and toss to coat. Cover and refrigerate for at least 1 hour.

Yield: 5 servings
Nutritional Analysis: One (¾ cup) serving equals 103 calories, 3 g fat, 15 g carbohydrate, 4 g protein
Diabetic Exchanges: 1 vegetable, ½ starch

Cilantro Lime Cod

4 cod fillets (2 pounds)
¼ teaspoon pepper

1 tablespoon dried minced onion
1 garlic clove, minced
1 tablespoon olive oil
1 teaspoon ground cumin
¼ cup minced fresh cilantro *or* parsley
2 limes, thinly sliced
1 tablespoon canola oil-based butter

Place each fillet on a 15-in. x 12-in. piece of heavy-duty foil. Sprinkle with pepper. In a small saucepan, sauté onion and garlic in oil; stir in cumin. Spoon over fillets; spinkle with cilantro. Place lime slices over each; drizzle with butter. Fold foil around fish and seal tightly. Place on a baking sheet. Bake at 375 degrees for 35-40 minutes or until fish flakes easily with a fork.

Yield: 8 servings
Nutritional Analysis: One serving equals 209 calories, 6 g fat, 3 g carbohydrate, 28 g protein
Diabetic Exchanges: 2 very lean meat, ½ fat

Chicken Burritos

¼ cup olive oil
¼ cup lime juice
4 garlic cloves, minced
1 tablespoon minced fresh parsley or 1 teaspoon dried parsley flakes
1 teaspoon ground cumin
1 teaspoon dried oregano
¼ teaspoon pepper
4 boneless skinless chicken breast halves (1 pound)
6 low-carb, fat-free flour tortillas
Shredded lettuce, diced tomatoes, and other vegetable condiments of your choice

In a large resealable plastic bag or shallow glass container, combine the first 7 ingredients. Add chicken and turn to coat. Seal or cover and refrigerate 8 hours or overnight, turning occasionally. Drain and discard marinade. Grill chicken, uncovered, over medium heat for 5-7 minutes on each side or until juices run clear. Cut into thin strips; serve in tortillas or taco shells with desired vegetable condiments.

Yield: 6 servings

Nutritional Analysis: One serving equals 201 calories, 5 g fat, 15 g carbohydrate, 24 g protein
Diabetic Exchanges: 3 lean meat, 1 starch, ½ fat

Lemon Chicken

½ cup water
¼ cup lemon juice
2 tablespoons dried minced onion
1 tablespoon dried parsley flakes
1 tablespoon Worcestershire sauce
1 garlic clove, minced
1 teaspoon dill seed
½ teaspoon curry powder
½ teaspoon pepper
8 boneless skinless chicken breast halves (2 pounds), cut up

In a large resealable bag or shallow glass container, combine the first 9 ingredients. Add chicken and turn to coat. Seal or cover and refrigerate for 4-6 hours. Drain and discard marinade. Grill chicken, covered, over low heat for 50-60 minutes or until juices run clear, turning several times.

Yield: 8 servings
Nutritional Analysis: One serving equals 156 calories, 4 g fat, 2 g carbohydrates, 28 g protein
Diabetic Exchanges: 3 lean meat

Cajun Salmon Steaks

2 salmon steaks (6 ounces, 1 inch thick)
½ teaspoon Worcestershire sauce
½ teaspoon lemon juice
½ teaspoon Cajun *or* Creole seasoning
½ cup diced green pepper
½ cup diced red pepper

Place the salmon in an ungreased 8-in. square microwave-safe dish. Rub with Worcestershire sauce and lemon juice; sprinkle with Cajun seasoning. Sprinkle peppers on top. Cover and microwave on high for 5-6 minutes, turning once, or until fish flakes easily with a fork. Let stand, covered, for 1 minute.

Yield: 2 servings
Nutritional Analysis: One serving equals 268 calories, 12 g fat, 4 g carbohydrate, 36 g protein
Diabetic Exchanges: 3 lean meat, 1 vegetable, 1 fat

Garlic Chicken

½ cup dry bread crumbs
¼ cup reduced-fat grated Parmesan cheese
2 tablespoons minced fresh parsley
¼ teaspoon pepper
¼ cup skim milk
6 boneless skinless chicken breast halves (1 ½ pounds)
¼ cup canola oil-based butter
2 garlic cloves, minced
2 tablespoons lemon juice
Pinch paprika

In a large resealable plastic bag, combine the first 5 ingredients. Place milk in a shallow bowl. Dip chicken in milk, then shake in the crumb mixture. Place in a greased 13-in. x 9-in. x 2-in. baking dish. Combine the butter, garlic, and lemon juice; drizzle over the chicken. Sprinkle with paprika. Bake, uncovered, at 350 degrees for 25-30 minutes.

Yield: 6 servings
Nutritional Analysis: One serving equals 172 calories, 6 g fat, 4 g carbohydrate, 30 g protein
Diabetic Exchanges: 3 lean meat, 1 fat, ½ starch

Chili Chicken Breasts

1 teaspoon chili powder
½ teaspoon ground cumin
¼ teaspoon garlic powder
¼ teaspoon cayenne pepper
4 boneless skinless chicken breast halves (1 pound)

1 teaspoon canola oil
¼ cup chopped green onions
1 jalapeno pepper, seeded and finely chopped
1 garlic clove, minced
1 can (14 1/2 ounces) diced tomatoes, undrained
1 teaspoon cornstarch
2 teaspoons water

Combine the first 4 ingredients, rub over chicken. In a nonstick skillet, brown chicken in oil on both sides. Add onions, jalapeno, and garlic; sauté for 1 minute. Add tomatoes; bring to a boil. Reduce heat; cover and simmer for 15-20 minutes. Remove chicken and keep warm. In a small bowl, combine cornstarch and water until smooth; stir in tomato mixture. Bring to a boil; cook and stir for 1 minute or until slightly thickened. Serve over chicken.

Yield: 4 servings
Nutritional Analysis: One serving equals 164 calories, 4 g fat, 4 g carbohydrate, 28 g protein
Diabetic Exchanges: 3 lean meat, 1 vegetable

Broccoli-Cabbage Slaw

2 cups shredded cabbage
2 cups broccoli florets
1 cup cauliflowerets
1 medium red onion, thinly sliced
¼ cup reduced-fat mayonnaise
¼ cup fat-free plain yogurt
¼ cup reduced-fat sour cream
¼ cup reduced-fat shredded Parmesan cheese

In a salad bowl, combine the cabbage, broccoli, cauliflower, and onion. In a small bowl, combine the remaining ingredients. Pour over vegetables and toss to coat. Cover and refrigerate until serving.

Yield: 6 servings
Nutritional Analysis: One (¾ cup) serving equals 116 calories, 6 g fat, 15 g carbohydrate, 5 g protein
Diabetic Exchanges: 1 vegetable, 1 fat, ½ starch

Herbed Lime Chicken

1 bottle (16 ounces) fat-free Italian salad dressing
½ cup lime juice
1 lime, halved and sliced
3 garlic cloves, minced
1 teaspoon dried thyme
8 boneless skinless chicken breast halves (2 pounds)

In a bowl, combine the first 5 ingredients. Remove ½ cup for basting; cover and refrigerate. Pour remaining marinade into a large resealable plastic bag; add chicken. Seal bag and turn to coat; refrigerate for 8-10 hours. Drain and discard marinade. Grill chicken, uncovered, over medium heat for 5 minutes. Turn chicken; baste with the reserved marinade. Grill 5-7 minutes longer, basting occasionally.

Yield: 8 servings
Nutritional Analysis: One serving equals 172 calories, 4 g fat, 6 g carbohydrate, 28 g protein
Diabetic Exchanges: 3 lean meat

Stuffed Sole

2 tablespoons canola oil-based butter
2 tablespoons lemon juice
½ teaspoon salt
¼ teaspoon pepper
1 package (10 ounces) frozen chopped broccoli, thawed and drained
1 cup cooked rice
1 cup (4 ounces) shredded reduced-fat cheddar cheese
8 sole *or* whitefish fillets (4 ounces each)
Paprika

In a small bowl, combine the butter, lemon juice, salt, and pepper. In another bowl, combine the broccoli, rice, cheese, and half of the butter mixture. Spoon ½ cup onto each fillet. Roll up and place seam side down in a baking dish coated with nonstick cooking spray. Pour remaining butter mixture over roll-ups. Bake, uncovered, at 350 degrees for 25 minutes or until fish flakes easily with a fork. Baste with pan drippings; sprinkle with paprika.

Yield: 8 servings

Nutritional Analysis: One serving equals 231 calories, 7 g fat, 12 g carbohydrate, 30 g protein
Diabetic Exchanges: 3 lean meat, 1 vegetable, ½ starch

Mushroom Spinach Tart

2 tablespoons seasoned bread crumbs
½ pound fresh mushrooms, sliced
½ cup chopped onion
1 tablespoon olive oil
1 package (10 ounces) frozen chopped spinach, thawed and squeezed dry
1 cup skim milk
1 cup egg substitute
¼ teaspoon salt
¼ teaspoon pepper
1 cup shredded reduced-fat Mexican cheese
½ cup grated reduced-fat Parmesan cheese

Coat a 9-in. pie plate with nonstick cooking spray. Sprinkle bottom and sides with bread crumbs; shake out the excess. Set plate aside. In a nonstick skillet, sauté mushrooms and onion in oil for 12-14 minutes or until all of the liquid has evaporated. Remove from the heat; stir in spinach. In a bowl, combine the milk, egg substitute, salt, and pepper. Stir in the spinach mixture, 1 cup Mexican cheese blend and Parmesan cheese. Pour into prepared pie plate. Bake at 350 degrees for 35-40 minutes or until a knife inserted near the center comes out clean. Sprinkle remaining cheese around edge of tart. Let stand for 5 minutes before slicing.

Yield: 8 servings
Nutritional Analysis: One piece equals 176 calories, 8 g fat, 10 g carbohydrate, 16 g protein
Diabetic Exchanges: 2 lean meat, 1 vegetable, 1 fat, ½ starch

LUNCHES

Garden Tuna Sandwiches

2 cans (6 ounces) water-packed tuna, drained
½ cup chopped peeled cucumber
½ shredded carrot
¼ cup finely chopped green onions
½ cup fat-free mayonnaise
¼ cup Dijon mustard
1 tablespoon fat-free sour cream
1 teaspoon lemon juice
¼ teaspoon pepper
8 slices whole wheat bread
4 lettuce leaves

In a bowl, combine the tuna, cucumber, carrot, onions, mayonnaise, mustard, sour cream, lemon juice, and pepper. Spread on four slices of bread; top with lettuce and remaining bread.

Yield: 4 servings
Nutritional Analysis: One sandwich equals 236 calories, 4 g fat, 32 g carbohydrate, 18 g protein
Diabetic Exchanges: 2 starch, 1 ½ lean meat, 1 vegetable

Mushroom Turkey Burger

2 pounds ground turkey breast
1 can (4 ounces) mushroom stems and pieces, drained
¼ cup egg substitute
½ cup chopped onion
¼ cup ketchup
1 teaspoon Italian seasoning
¼ teaspoon pepper
¼ teaspoon Worcestershire sauce

In a bowl, combine all ingredients. Divide into 8 patties and grill, covered, over medium heat until meat is no longer pink, turning once.

Yield: 8 servings
Nutritional Analysis: One serving equals 186 calories, 6 g fat, 4 g carbohydrate, 29 g protein
Diabetic Exchanges: 3 lean meat, 1 vegetable

Chicken Cheddar Wraps

½ cup (4 ounces) fat-free sour cream
¾ cup chunky salsa
2 tablespoons light mayonnaise
4 boneless skinless chicken breast halves (1 pound)
1 cup (4 ounces) fat-free shredded cheddar cheese
½ cup thinly sliced fresh mushrooms
2 cups shredded lettuce
6 low-carb, fat-free flour tortillas
Tomato wedges

In a bowl, combine the sour cream, salsa, and mayonnaise. Stir in chicken, cheese, and mushrooms. Divide lettuce between tortillas. Place about ½ cup chicken mixture on each tortilla. Fold sides over the fillings. Garnish with tomato.

Yield: 6 wraps
Nutritional Analysis: One wrap equals 167 calories, 3 g fat, 17 g carbohydrate, 18 g protein
Diabetic Exchanges: 1 starch, 2 lean meat, 1 vegetable

Vegetarian Burritos

10 egg whites (or equivalent egg substitute)
¼ teaspoon pepper
1 cup salsa
¼ cup chopped onion
1 cup (4 ounces) fat-free shredded cheddar cheese
8 low-carb, fat-free flour tortillas

In a bowl, beat the eggs and pepper. Pour into a skillet that has been coated with nonstick cooking spray. Cook and stir over medium heat until eggs are partially set. Add salsa and onion, cook, and stir until eggs are completely set. Sprinkle with cheese. Spoon about ½ cup down the center of each tortilla; fold ends and sides over filling. Serve immediately.

Yield: 8 servings
Nutritional Analysis: One serving equals 146 calories, 2 g fat, 20 g carbohydrate, 12 g protein
Diabetic Exchanges: 1 starch, 1 vegetable, 1 lean meat

Italian Mushroom Salad

2 pounds fresh mushrooms, quartered
3 medium tomatoes, cut into wedges
1 cup fat-free Italian salad dressing
1 teaspoon dried parsley flakes
½ teaspoon garlic powder
¼ cup chopped onion
½ teaspoon dried basil
3 cups fresh spinach leaves
4 turkey bacon strips, cooked and chopped

Place mushrooms and tomatoes in a large shallow dish. Combine the next 5 ingredients; drizzle over mushrooms and tomatoes. Cover and refrigerate overnight, stirring once. Line a serving platter or bowl with spinach. Using a slotted spoon, arrange vegetables over spinach. Sprinkle with turkey bacon.

Yield: 8 servings
Nutritional Analysis: One (1 cup) serving equals 37 calories, 1 g fat 8 g carbohydrate, 1 g protein
Diabetic Exchanges: 1 vegetable

Soft Chicken Tacos

4 boneless skinless chicken breast halves (1 pound), cut into cubes
1 can (15 ounces) black beans, rinsed and drained
1 cup salsa
1 tablespoon taco seasoning
½ cup fat-free sour cream
6 low-carb, fat-free flour tortillas
Optional Toppings: shredded lettuce, fat-free shredded cheddar cheese, diced tomatoes, and sliced green onions.

In a skillet that has been coated with nonstick cooking spray, cook chicken until juices run clear. Add beans, salsa, and taco seasoning; heat through. Remove from heat and add sour cream. Spoon the chicken mixture down the center of each tortillas. Garnish with toppings of your choice.

Yield: 6 servings
Nutritional Analysis: One taco equals 196 calories, 4 g fat, 18 g carbohydrate, 22 g protein
Diabetic Exchanges: 1 starch, 2 lean meat

Spinach Chicken Wraps

1 package (10 ounces) fresh spinach
½ cup chopped fresh mushrooms
1 green onion, finely chopped
1 garlic cloves, minced
1 tablespoon olive oil
2 egg whites, lightly beaten
¼ cup crumbled feta cheese
¼ cup dry bread crumbs
¼ teaspoon dried rosemary, crushed
4 boneless skinless chicken breast halves (1 pound)
½ teaspoon dried basil
½ teaspoon dried thyme
¼ teaspoon pepper
4 low-carb, fat-free flour tortilla wraps

In a large saucepan, place spinach in a steamer basket over 1 in. of boiling water. Cover and steam for 2-3 minutes or just until wilted. When cool enough to handle, squeeze spinach dry and finely chop. In a nonstick skillet, sauté the mushrooms, onion, and garlic in oil until tender. Add spinach; cook and stir for 2 minutes. Transfer to a bowl. Add egg whites, cheese, and bread crumbs, mix well. Flatten chicken to ¼-in. thickness. Combine basil, thyme, and pepper; rub over one side of chicken. Spread spinach mixture over wraps and roll up. Secure with toothpicks. In a large saucepan, place wraps in a steamer basket over 1 in. of boiling water. Cover and steam for 12-15 minutes or until chicken is no longer pink.

Yield: 4 servings

Nutritional Analysis: One serving equals 238 calories, 6 g fat, 16 g carbohydrate, 30 g protein
Diabetic Exchanges: 2 lean meat, 1 vegetable, 1 fat

Broccoli Cheddar Soup

1 large bunch broccoli, coarsely chopped (5 cups)
2 tablespoons cornstarch
2 cups skim milk
1 cup chicken broth
1 tablespoon canola oil-based butter
¼ teaspoon salt
1/8 teaspoon pepper
1 cup (8 ounces) shredded fat-free cheddar cheese
Dash paprika

In a saucepan, bring 1 inch of water to a boil. Place broccoli in a steamer basket over water. Cover and steam for 5-8 minutes or until crisp-tender. Meanwhile, in another saucepan, combine the cornstarch, milk, and broth until smooth. Bring to a boil, cook, and stir for 2 minutes or until thickened. Stir in the butter, salt, and pepper. Reduce heat. Add cheese and broccoli; heat just until cheese is melted. Sprinkle with paprika.

Yield: 4 servings
Nutritional Analysis: One serving equals 123 calories, 3 g fat, 17 g carbohydrate, 7 g protein
Diabetic Exchanges: 2 vegetable, 1 lean meat, 1 fat

BREAKFAST

Oat Waffles

1 cup all-purpose flour
1 cup oat flour
4 teaspoons baking powder
3 egg whites
1 ¾ cups skim milk
2 tablespoons canola oil
1 teaspoon vanilla extract

In a bowl, combine the first 3 ingredients. Combine the egg whites, milk, oil, and vanilla; stir into dry ingredients just until combined. Pour batter by ½ cupfuls into a preheated waffle iron; bake until golden brown.

Yield: 8 waffles
Nutritional Analysis: One waffle equals 147 calories, 3 g fat, 24 g carbohydrate, 6 g protein
Diabetic Exchanges: 1 ½ starch

Country Scrambled Eggs

12 egg whites, 2 yolks
¾ cup diced fully cooked ham
¾ cup fat-free shredded cheddar cheese
½ cup chopped fresh mushrooms
¼ cup chopped onion

In a bowl, beat eggs. Add ham, cheese, mushrooms, and onion. Lightly coat skillet with cooking spray; add egg mixture. Cook and stir over medium heat until eggs are completely set and cheese is melted.

Yield: 4 servings
Nutritional Analysis: One serving equals 134 calories, 6 g fat, 4 g carbohydrate, 16 g protein
Diabetic Exchanges: ½ vegetable, 1 fat, 1 ½ lean meats

Veggie Omelet

¼ cup diced green pepper
¼ cup diced onion
¼ cup sliced mushrooms
4 egg whites
Pinch pepper
2 tablespoons fat-free shredded cheddar cheese

In an 8-in. skillet, sauté green pepper, onion, and mushrooms in cooking spray until tender. Remove and set aside. In a small bowl, beat egg whites, salt, and pepper. Pour into a skillet. Cook over medium heat; as eggs set, lift edges, letting uncooked portion flow underneath. When the eggs are set, spoon vegetables and cheese over one side; fold omelet over filling. Cover and let stand for 1-2 minutes or until cheese is melted.

Yield: 1 serving
Nutritional Analysis: One serving equals 98 calories, 2 g fat, 3 g carbohydrate, 17 g protein
Diabetic Exchanges: 1 vegetable, 2 lean protein

Cheese Omelet

4 egg whites
¼ teaspoon onion powder
¼ teaspoon dried basil
¼ teaspoon dried parsley flakes
¼ teaspoon celery seed
¼ cup fat-free shredded cheddar cheese

In a bowl, beat egg whites and seasonings. Lightly coat skillet with cooking spray. Add egg mixture; cook over medium heat. As eggs set, lift edges, letting uncooked portion flow underneath. When eggs are completely set, remove from the heat. Place cheese over half of the eggs. Fold in half and serve.

Yield: 1 serving
Nutritional Analysis: One serving equals 118 calories, 2 g fat, 6 g carbohydrate, 19 g protein
Diabetic Exchanges: 1 vegetable, 2 lean protein

Dilly Scrambled Eggs

6 egg whites, 2 yolks
¼ cup skim milk
Dash pepper
1 teaspoon snipped fresh dill *or* ¼ teaspoon dill weed

In a bowl, beat the eggs, milk, and pepper. Lightly coat skillet with cooking spray; add egg mixture. Cook and stir gently over medium heat until eggs are almost set. Sprinkle with cheese and dill; cook until eggs are completely set and cheese is melted.

Yield: 2 servings
Nutritional Analysis: One serving equals 139 calories, 7 g fat, 3 g carbohydrate, 16 g protein
Diabetic Exchanges: 1 fat, 2 lean protein

Spinach Egg Bake

1 cup seasoned bread crumbs
2 packages (10 ounces *each*) frozen chopped spinach, thawed and squeezed dry
3 cups (24 ounces) small-curd, fat-free cottage cheese
½ cup grated fat-free Parmesan cheese
8 egg whites, 2 yolks

Sprinkle ¼ cup bread crumbs into a cooking spray-coated 8-in. square baking dish. Bake at 350 degrees for 3-5 minutes or until golden brown. In a bowl, combine the spinach, cottage cheese, Parmesan cheese, six egg whites, one yolk, and remaining crumbs. Spread over the baked crumbs. Beat remaining eggs; pour over spinach mixture. Bake uncovered at 350 degrees for 45 minutes or until a knife inserted near the center comes out clean. Let stand for 5-10 minutes before serving.

Yield: 4 servings
Nutritional Analysis: One serving equals 176 calories, 4 g fat, 15 g carbohydrate, 20 g protein
Diabetic Exchanges: 2 lean meat, 1 starch, 1 vegetable, 1 fat

DESSERTS

Creamy Raspberry Pie

1 package (3 ounces) sugar-free raspberry gelatin
½ cup boiling water
1 cup fat-free frozen vanilla yogurt
1 cup fresh *or* frozen unsweetened raspberries
¼ cup lime juice
2 cups fat-free whipped topping
1 reduced-fat graham cracker crust (9 inches)
Lime slices and additional raspberries and whipped topping, optional

In a bowl, dissolve the gelatin in boiling water. Stir in frozen yogurt until melted. Add raspberries and lime juice. Fold in whipped topping. Spoon into crust. Refrigerate for 3 hours or until firm. Garnish with lime, raspberries, and whipped topping.

Yield: 8 servings
Nutritional Analysis: One slice equals 86 calories, 2 g fat, 13 g carbohydrate, 4 g protein
Diabetic Exchanges: 1 starch, ½ fruit

Cherry Cream Pie

4 ounces fat-free cream cheese, softened
1 ½ cups sugar-free cherry pie filing
2 cups fat-free whipped topping
1 reduced-fat graham cracker crust (9 inches)

In a mixing bowl, beat cream cheese until smooth. Fold in the pie filling and whipped topping until blended. Spoon into crust. Cover and freeze for 8 hours or overnight. Remove from the freezer 15 minutes before serving.

Yield: 8 servings
Nutritional Analysis: One piece equals 94 calories, 2 g fat, 15 g carbohydrate, 4 g protein
Diabetic Exchanges: 1 starch, ½ fruit

Lemon Mousse

¼ cup sugar
Sugar substitute, such as Splenda or Stevia, equivalent to ½ cup sugar
½ cup cornstarch
3 cups skim milk
2/3 cup lemon juice
1 ½ teaspoons grated lemon peel
¼ teaspoon vanilla extract
2 cups fat-free whipped topping

In a saucepan, combine the sugar, sugar substitute, and cornstarch; gradually stir in milk until smooth. Bring to a boil over medium heat, stirring constantly. Cook and stir for 2 minutes or until thickened and bubbly. Remove from the heat. Stir in lemon juice, peel, and vanilla. Set saucepan in ice; stir until mixture reaches room temperature, about 5 minutes. Fold in whipped topping. Spoon into dessert dishes. Refrigerate for at least 1 hour before serving.

Yield: 10 servings
Nutritional Analysis: One (½ cup) serving equals 61 calories, 1 g fat, 10 g carbohydrate, 3 g protein
Diabetic Exchanges: 1 starch, 1 fruit

Pear Squares

1 ½ pounds pears, sliced
3 tablespoon all-purpose flour
¼ cup unsweetened apple juice concentrate
¾ cup reduced-fat graham cracker crumbs (about 10 squares)
½ teaspoon ground cinnamon
Dash ground nutmeg
2 tablespoons canola oil-based stick butter
½ cup fat-free whipped topping
Additional ground cinnamon

In a bowl, toss the pears, 1 tablespoon flour, and apple juice concentrate. Spoon into an 8-in. square baking dish coated with nonstick cooking spray. In a bowl, combine the crumbs, cinnamon, nutmeg, and remaining flour. Cut in butter until mixture resembles coarse crumbs. Sprinkle over pears.

Bake at 375 degrees for 30 minutes or until pears are tender and topping is lightly browned. Serve warm or chilled. Cut into squares; top with whipped topping and cinnamon.

Yield: 9 servings
Nutritional Analysis: One serving equals 128 calories, 4 g fat, 22 g carbohydrate, 1 g protein
Diabetic Exchanges: 1 starch, ½ fruit, ½ fat

Eggnog Pudding

2 cups skim milk
1 package (3.4 ounces) sugar-free instant vanilla pudding mix
½ teaspoon ground nutmeg
¼ teaspoon rum extract
Additional nutmeg, optional

In a bowl, combine the first 4 ingredients. Beat for 2 minutes. Spoon into individual dishes. Chill. Sprinkle with nutmeg if desired.

Yield: 4 servings
Nutritional Analysis: One (½ cup) serving equals 101 calories, 1 g fat, 16 g carbohydrate, 7 g protein.
Diabetic Exchanges: 1 starch, ½ lean meat

Orange Whip

1 can (11 ounces) mandarin oranges, drained
1 cup (8 ounces) fat-free, low-carb vanilla yogurt
2 tablespoons orange juice concentrate
2 cups fat-free whipped topping

In a bowl, combine the oranges, yogurt, and orange juice concentrate. Fold in the whipped topping. Spoon into serving dishes. Cover and freeze until firm. Remove from the freezer 20 minutes before serving.

Yield: 4 servings
Nutritional Analysis: One (¾ cup) serving equals 81 calories, 1 g fat, 15 g carbohydrate, 3 g protein
Diabetic Exchanges: 1 fruit, 1 starch

Blueberry Pie

¼ cup sugar
Sugar substitute, such as Splenda or Stevia, equivalent to ¼ cup sugar
2 tablespoons cornstarch
¾ cup water
4 cups fresh *or* frozen blueberries, thawed
1 reduced-fat graham cracker crust (9 inches)
Fat-free whipped topping

In a saucepan, combine sugar and cornstarch. Stir in water until smooth. Bring to a boil over medium heat, cook and stir for 2 minutes. Add blueberries. Cook for 3 minutes, stirring occasionally. Pour into crust. Chill. Garnish with whipped topping.

Yield: 8 servings
Nutritional Analysis: One piece equals 94 calories, 2 g fat, 17 g carbohydrate, 2 g protein
Diabetic Exchanges: 1 starch, 1 fruit

Light Carrot Cake

Sugar substitute equivalent to ¼ cup sugar
1 tablespoon canola oil
½ cup sugar-free apple sauce
1/3 cup orange juice concentrate
3 egg whites
1 cup all-purpose flour
1 teaspoon baking powder
1 teaspoon ground cinnamon
½ teaspoon ground allspice
¼ teaspoon baking soda
1 cup grated carrots
2 teaspoons confectioners' sugar

In a mixing bowl, combine the first 5 ingredients; beat for 30 seconds. Combine flour, baking powder, cinnamon, allspice, and baking soda; add to the orange juice mixture and mix well. Stir in carrots. Pour into an 8-in. square baking pan that has been coated with nonstick cooking spray. Bake at 350 degrees for 30 minutes or until a toothpick inserted near the center comes out clean. Cool; dust with confectioners' sugar.

Yield: 9 servings

Nutritional Analysis: One serving equals 147 calories, 3 g fat, 27 g carbohydrate, 3 g protein
Diabetic Exchanges: 2 starch, ½ fat

Chocolate Mousse

¾ cup skim milk
1 package (1.4 ounces) sugar-free instant chocolate pudding mix
½ cup fat-free sour cream
3 ounces fat-free cream cheese, cubed
½ teaspoon vanilla extract
1 carton (8 ounces) fat-free whipped topping
1 tablespoon chocolate cookie crumbs

In a bowl, whisk milk and pudding mix for 2 minutes (mixture will be very thick). In a mixing bowl, beat the sour cream, cream cheese, and vanilla. Add pudding; mix well. Fold in whipped topping. Spoon into individual dishes. Sprinkle with cookie crumbs. Refrigerate until serving.

Yield: 6 servings
Nutritional Analysis: One serving equals 106 calories, 2 g fat, 18 g carbohydrate, 4 g protein
Diabetic Exchanges: 1 ½ starch

Lemon Blueberry Cheesecake

1 package (3 ounces) sugar-free lemon gelatin
1 cup boiling water
2 tablespoons canola oil-based butter
1 tablespoon canola oil
1 cup reduced-fat graham cracker crumbs (about 16 squares)
1 carton (24 ounces) fat-free cottage cheese
¼ cup sugar
Sugar substitute equivalent to ¼ cup sugar
TOPPING:
Sugar substitute equivalent to 2 tablespoons sugar
1 ½ teaspoons cornstarch
¼ cup water
1 ½ cups fresh *or* frozen blueberries
1 teaspoon lemon juice

In a bowl, dissolve gelatin in boiling water; cool. Combine butter and oil; add crumbs and blend well. Press onto the bottom of a 9-in. springform pan. Chill. In a blender, process cottage cheese, sugar substitute, and sugar until smooth. While processing, slowly add cooled gelatin. Pour into crust; chill overnight.

For topping, combine sugar substitute and cornstarch in a saucepan; stir in water until smooth. Add 1 cup blueberries. Bring to a boil; cook and stir for 2 minutes or until thickened. Stir in lemon juice; cool slightly. Process in a blender until smooth. Refrigerate until completely cooled. Carefully run a knife around edge of pan to loosen cheesecake; remove sides of pan. Spread the blueberry mixture over the top. Top with remaining blueberries.

Yield: 12 servings
Nutritional Analysis: One piece equals 156 calories, 4 g fat, 22 g carbohydrate, 8 g protein
Diabetic Exchanges: 1 ½ starch, ½ fruit, ½ fat

No-Bake Chocolate Cheesecake

¾ cup reduced-fat graham cracker crumbs (about 12 squares)
2 tablespoons canola oil-based butter
1 envelope unflavored gelatin
1 cup cold water
4 squares (1 ounce *each*) semisweet chocolate, coarsely chopped
4 packages (8 ounces *each*) fat-free cream cheese
Sugar substitute equivalent to 1 cup sugar
¼ cup sugar
¼ cup baking cocoa
2 teaspoons vanilla extract
TOPPING:
2 cups fresh raspberries
1 ounce white candy coating

In a bowl, combine cracker crumbs and butter; press onto the bottom of a 9-in. spring form pan. Bake at 375 degrees for 8-10 minutes or until lightly browning. Cool on a wire rack. For filling, in a small saucepan, sprinkle gelatin over cold water; let stand for 1 minute. Heat over low heat, stirring until gelatin is completely dissolved. Add the semisweet chocolate; stir until melted. In a mixing bowl, beat the cream cheese, sugar substitute, and sugar until smooth. Gradually add the chocolate mixture and cocoa. Beat in vanilla. Pour into crust; refrigerate for 2-3 hours or until firm. Arrange raspberries on top of cheesecake.

In a heavy saucepan or microwave, melt white candy coating; stir until smooth. Drizzle or pipe over berries. Carefully run a knife around edge of pan to loosen. Remove sides of pan.

Yield: 12 servings
Nutritional Analysis: One slice equals 158 calories, 6 g fat, 27 g carbohydrate, 9 g protein
Diabetic Exchanges: 2 starch, 1 lean meat, 1 fat

Pumpkin Spice Dip

1 package (8 ounces) fat-free cream cheese
½ cup canned pumpkin
Sugar substitute equivalent to ½ cup sugar
1 teaspoon ground cinnamon
1 teaspoon vanilla extract
1 teaspoon maple flavoring
½ teaspoon pumpkin pie spice
½ teaspoon ground nutmeg
1 carton (8 ounces) fat-free whipped topping

In a large mixing bowl, combine the cream cheese, pumpkin, and sugar substitute; mix well. Beat in the cinnamon, vanilla, maple flavoring, pumpkin pie spice, and nutmeg. Fold in whipped topping. Refrigerate until serving.

Yield: 4 cups
Nutritional Analysis: One serving (3 tablespoons) equals 33 calories, 1 g fat, 4 g carbohydrate, 1 g protein
Diabetic Exchanges: ½ starch

Peanut Butter Pudding

2 cups skim milk
4 tablespoons reduced-fat creamy peanut butter
1 package (1 ounce) sugar-free instant vanilla pudding mix
½ cup fat-free whipped topping
4 teaspoons chocolate syrup

In a bowl, whisk the milk and peanut butter until blended. Add pudding mix, whisk for 2 minutes or until slightly thickened. Spoon into dessert dishes. Refrigerate for at least 5 minutes or until set. Just before serving, dollop with shipped topping and drizzle with chocolate syrup.

Yield: 4 servings
Nutritional Analysis: One serving equals 172 calories, 8 g fat, 17 g carbohydrate, 8 g protein
Diabetic Exchanges: 1 starch, 1 lean meat, 1 fat

CHAPTER EIGHT KEY POINTS

- 1) The right foods in the right amounts should be your focus.
- 2) You can construct fancy recipes, but this is unnecessary. Be creative and plan ahead using foods you like.
- 3) Did I mention "be creative"?

CHAPTER NINE

THE PSYCHOLOGY OF SUCCESS

Okay, here it comes. We were almost tempted not to write this chapter. The subject of food and how we consume it could occupy either one sentence or a two-volume textbook. However, we believe this needs to be addressed to the best of our abilities, no matter how difficult the subject matter.

The fascinating thing is the variety of personal backgrounds that often bring people to the same place. A study of the microcosm of the individual authors can tell you that. Joe came from a family background where health was not as much of a priority. Obesity and smoking ran rampant. Part of his make-up is to be driven to avoid some of the same mistakes he had seen time and again.

My parents quit smoking in their forties, took up jogging, and co-founded a local runners club. I couldn't help some of their enthusiasm rubbing off on me. I did distance running throughout grade school and into high school. My parents were somewhat rigid about food, which led me to rebel in college. I turned my back on running and healthy eating, and ultimately had to go pay Joe a lot of money to try to get my girlish figure back.

Two different approaches and two different outcomes. Of course, we all know of people who have followed their parents' good examples or poor examples their entire lives. My point is this: no matter what your background, you have to start at this moment in time. Although your environment, upbringing, and psychological make-up may color your approach, you will have to start by wiping the slate clean and going forward from here. The parental/spouse/fill-in-the-blank blame game ends now. As we all know, a similar environment may produce an Olympic quality athlete or a broken person with a 50-inch waistline. Even if our parents all had Ph.D.'s in psychology, they still wouldn't get it right all the time. We have known individuals who believe a single comment at a critical point in life contributes to anorexia or other problems. However, as adults, we choose what goes into our mouths. We control what goes into our body. No one else can influence that other than us, right? But after a while, who or what has control—us or our ever-expanding waistline? What we choose to eat and drink is intensely personal, and we are often more reluctant to talk about it than even politics or religion. The reality is that we cannot live in a state of rebellion and a state of health simultaneously. We can't come into your house and pry open your mouth with the "Jaws of Life" and pour some sprouts down your throat. You will have to choose today how you will live. "I'm trying," cannot be an excuse for not doing.

All of us have had maladaptive ways of dealing with food at one time or another, and it's only when it becomes more extreme that it becomes a problem. I believe the majority of people who are not eating healthy are spending the bulk of their time in either denial or rationalization. Deep down we know what we are doing is bad for us, but we simply chose to ignore it. If your eating is a significant problem or causes severe stress, you should really be getting more detailed help. Counseling is a relationship over time, and not fully within the scope of any book. A therapeutic counseling relationship is worthwhile and should be undertaken with earnest for those who need it. If you bought this book you are already trying to move out of denial and I commend you. Let's move on to creating new habits and developing discipline for a lifetime.

Patience is a Virtue

This is by far the most important part of any weight-loss or fitness program. You must learn to not only emphasize your strengths but also confront and overcome your weaknesses. Losing weight will be work; there is no way around that. However, with a good program like this, it is not an overwhelming amount of work. And for that matter, when did we as Americans become afraid of work? We built this country, built the space shuttle, and, heck, our kids play games on computers more sophisticated than what put Armstrong on the moon (Neil, not Lance). Why are we unwilling to work on our health? We work hard; we have everything imaginable to play hard. We even take our lemonade hard—just ask Mike. But when it comes to our health, we are a generation sticking our tongues out at physical well-being. I used to do it too. Is anything that's worthwhile ever very easy? Of course not. It is a lifelong commitment. My father always said, "Patience is a virtue." It used to drive me nuts as a kid, but patience and persistence are unbelievably valuable as you approach a project such as this. I am also pleased to say that I am currently driving my eleven-year-old son nuts with that same phrase. My wife gave me a great example of this concept. She was frustrated that her progress seemed to be very slow. However when we looked at her progress over the months we found that her "set point" was getting lower and lower. She was 10 pounds lighter for several weeks, then 13 pounds lighter, and then later she was 16 pounds lighter. Although it took months, she was continuing to move forward.

Nothing sends me from zero to crazy faster than when I am trying to talk to a patient about diet and exercise and I get the dismissive wave of the hand and the patient says, "I already know what I need to do. I just need to do it." If you did, you would have already done it! It is time to get real and do some serious self-examination. For those of you who would rather have a root canal than discuss these types of things, guess again. The unexamined life is not worth living. (Someone once said that. Was it Thoreau? Emerson? Letterman?) Also, for those of you who think you always take responsibility for yourself and you really don't need a lot of outside help—there's something here for you too.

Take the Time

As you start this process, I want you to take a little time by yourself with no distractions. I mean totally no distractions. Turn the television off, put the kids in bed, and find the remote for your spouse so you have a few minutes of total privacy. Think about why you want to lose weight and get in shape. Put down all the reasons on paper. Also, jot down your personal strengths and weaknesses. What were your dieting failures in the past and what led to your dieting collapse? Get it done in one day. Don't let this self-analysis drag on for days and lead to paralysis. Finally, I want you to take all that stuff and shred it. That's right, rip it up and dance on top of it. Laugh, cry, or spit if you need to, but tear it up. Don't tape it up on your mirror for motivation. Your memory already knows what you did right and wrong in the past. That was the past, this is now. You are not a "loser" or a "failure" because of past problems. You are now a full-time student of nutrition and few students ever get 100% on every test. However, at the end of the course, you will be a lot smarter than when you started. Whether you are in denial or rationalization mode, you simply need to be honest with yourself, acknowledge that fact, and move forward. For those of you that are anal-retentive and like making lists, save it for your daily food logs.

Start at this point in time. If you truly can't leave the baggage behind, then get serious help for your mind as well as your body and see a counselor. The baggy clothes and the candy bar stuffed behind the flour canister aren't fooling anyone. And how much does food really comfort us when we are staring at the results in the mirror and riding the guilt and shame train? It is an "acceptable drug," but it is a destructive coping mechanism. It's that simple. Food will kill you just as dead as drugs, alcohol, or tobacco. Face it.

Metabolic Transformation in Action

>   Weighing myself is an exciting experience and I love going to stores to find new jeans or bathing suits! All this is a dream come true for me, a person with a lifelong track record of disordered eating and dieting. Today, I look and feel better at 40 than I ever have in my life! That's how it is with Metabolic Transformation.
>
>   On my own, I was fighting a losing battle. I am not immune to the psychologically charged nature of food and eating in this culture. We celebrate our victories and sooth our losses all with food. The pressure on women and girls to be "small and skinny" makes that struggle even harder. I am a large framed woman: I am 5'10" and wear a size 11 shoe! So "small and skinny" is not in the cards for me. However, since high school I made sad attempts to control my size that resulted in extreme disordered eating. My life revolved around dieting and the number on the scale. I hated my body. I tried every quick fix and popular diet you can think of. I would commence each program thinking, "This is the one," only to gain fat in the end. These popular diets also exaggerated the psychopathology behind my negative body image and disordered eating. My weight fluctuated, as did my dress size. I had no balance in my life and it negatively impacted upon important relationships. My unhealthy dealings with food were no more than an exercise in futility.
>
>   After working closely with Dr. Joe I have learned I can be slender, athletic, and lean! His program gives me the proper tools to do just this; there is no guesswork. My metabolism is ramped up, my lean body mass is stable, and my fat-burning capacity is full speed. As a result, disordered eating has vanished and I have carved out the body of a professional athlete. One of the greatest benefits is that I have maintained this for years now. I've even learned to handle events that arise like holidays, reunions, or other emotionally charged occasions. Accordingly, his numbers work the way he says they will work. He takes every pound on my body as seriously as if it was his own.
>
>   Most importantly I finally have both a healthy relationship with food and balance around eating. I can be present and "in the moment" with my daughter and husband, and not always worried about weight. I am finally enjoying my life, my family, and taking pride in my body!
>
>   Never did I think that I would be a competitive athlete after 40; I am! Never did I dream of having balance in my life with food; I do! The notion
>
>   continued ⟶

Metabolic Transformation in Action

> of eating normally without fear, disorder, and fat gain was a dream; it's come true! Thank you Dr. Joe, for your continued support, guidance, and believing in me. I owe my success to you!
>
> After
>
> Mary

The biggest reason to understand nutrition and exercise is your health. It is that straightforward and it never needs to get any more complicated than that. Looking better, playing more with your kids, or impressing the new girl at the office are all nice by-products of being in shape (unless of course you are married, in which case trying to impress the new girl at the office will get you a lot of couch time at home without a psychiatrist. In that scenario you probably need our next book, *Pot Bellies and the Sociopaths Who Love Them*. That will come next right after our vitamin book or before our cookbook. Maybe it's before our nutritional text for pets; I can never remember).

Health needs to be a big part of your goal. We have all failed at diets or other forms of discipline in our lives at one time or another. We can all hear the little devils that sit on our shoulders whispering how we cannot do something and how much we have failed in the past. It doesn't matter. This time I only want you to focus on one goal and say this to yourself: I want to learn about nutrition and exercise to improve my health for the rest of my life. I know you'll enjoy and revel in how you look when you're leaner and people start saying, "Hey! Are you working out? You look so much younger!" I want to make sure you're grounded in the long-term "why" of your metabolic transformation. I will come back to this single goal again at the end of the chapter. It is that important.

Girls (and Boys) Just Want to Have Fun

I believe that some of our problems with eating and our ignorance in the area of nutrition are simply because we have to have self-control or discipline in so many other areas that we want to have some chaos or fun in our dietary lives. Let's face it; food is neither illegal nor immoral, at least at this point anyway. Unfortunately that pursuit of "fun with food" can destroy our life span. As you decrease your carbohydrate intake, you will notice that high-sugar foods won't taste as good. Ex-smokers say the same about cigarettes. It doesn't mean that they don't want one, but they can use that change in taste to their advantage the same way you can with high-sugar foods. Do *not* try to force yourself to learn how to like those types of foods again. The loss of that pleasure may be a little disappointing at first, but I believe that you can replace that disappointment with the wonderful feelings of confidence and athleticism that will allow you to enjoy other areas of life that are not food related. I now love walking the golf course with my son no matter what the temperature.

I'll give you an example: previously, I would go to parties and as soon as I entered the gathering I was thinking about where the buffet table was located, when the meal would be served, and worrying that if I was at the end of the line that there wouldn't be enough to eat. Now I can spend time with my loved ones and friends and focus on catching up on their lives and sharing laughs and good times instead of worrying about food. Now I don't mind being at the back of the line!

Also, you will notice that high-fat or high-sugar foods will hurt your stomach when you aren't used to them. Learn that feeling—your body is telling you something. Listen to it! In fact, you will enjoy certain foods more since you won't be eating them as often and you will appreciate them. You'll enjoy those foods with a great sense of satisfaction during your "splurge meal" knowing you sacrificed and truly "earned" it.

Well, Excuuuuuse Me!

The key is that you cannot accept excuses or rationalizations from yourself. Now I'm not talking about slip-ups or mistakes because even the most dedicated of us will have a bad day. I'm talking about letting that bad meal turn into a bad day or week or . . . you get the picture. You don't have to trick yourself because you don't have anything to prove to anyone else. There's no particular goal to reach other than a better level of health and fitness.

We are all stressed, overworked, and pressed for time. You know what? So were our parents and grandparents. The major difference is they understood that hard work and sacrifice were just parts of daily living. They didn't have the money to reward themselves with a treat every time they did something like actually showing up for work and doing the job they were expected to do. One recent commercial shows the guy rewarding himself with a soda just for opening a jar of pickles!

Getting up every day and doing the things we are supposed to do is a decent and honorable thing. However, we don't need to reward ourselves by poisoning our bodies with junk food or portions so big our grandmother could have fed her entire big, fat Greek family plus the nice couple next door from one restaurant entrée. We don't need to sit and idly watch as our insurance premiums and co-pays go through the roof and our hard-earned cash flies out the door due to the complications of obesity. And it doesn't matter what age you are. I have seen people in their 70's and 80's benefit from this program. You are never too old to learn about good nutrition. Stress will follow you your entire life so you need to get rid of the idea of "stress eating" or soon the pounds will be following you. Stress eating needs to become a foreign concept instead of a daily occurrence.

Being "busy" to me is a lousy excuse, and one that I hear all the time. People will tell me that they are too busy, and when I discuss with them how they can eat healthy it's always the same: poor eye contact, nodding the head in agreement. I know that they are just humoring me. If you have time to stop at the fast food place or any type of grocery store then you are not "too busy." What you did, however, was make poor choices. Even the convenience store has something healthy. You can order the chicken sandwich, side salad, and water or the burger, fries, and a large Coke. It's your choice. Your vocal cords can speak either set of words. But you are more like Gollum in *The Lord of the Rings* saying, "Me wants it! Me needs it!" Then we'll see you out in the parking lot ripping into that raw burrito with your teeth. Think about it *before* you are faced with those situations. Say, "Chicken, my precious." You can do it.

It's ironic that times of prosperity can be problematic too. We give ourselves too much of a pat on the back for a job well done and think, "Ah, I can start again next week," or "I've earned it. Why do I need to bother?" Stress or no stress, we have to be on guard.

As Joe mentioned, too many of us want to blame our metabolism for lack of weight loss. Metabolism is indeed the key. It is not to be blamed when we understand how to operate in the appropriate macronutritional range. It is the key to losing body fat and maintaining your healthy new weight. If you haven't consumed enough nutrients, your metabolism will slow dramatically and you will have to work much longer and harder to lose weight. If you have consumed too much, you will gain weight. Too many of us blame our metabolism, but chips and a six-pack have nothing to do with a "slow metabolism." The excuse list could go on for pages, but none of them are valid. Focus on nutrition, discipline, health, and fun instead of the next creative rationalization.

Are You Looking at Me?

How many of us waste days or even years internalizing? It's not a pretty place at times. We must be willingly to accept responsibility for our poor dietary and exercise choices. However, we may be locked in our own minds of denial, unwilling to ask for help. "I can't lose weight, my metabolism is too slow." "My genes are bad." "I like the way I look. Why can't people accept me the way I am?" "I can always get back to the way I looked before." "I know what I need to do. I don't need the Diet Docs." Hey, hey, hey! Just a minute there, little mister.

We are not powerless over ourselves. At times it feels like we are looking down at ourselves and saying, "Hey, who's that fat guy who took my seat? He doesn't belong there, but he doesn't seem to be hurting or bothering anybody. I don't think I can move him. I guess I'll just leave him alone." And we walk away instead of saying, "Hey you! Yeah, you with your Big Gulp and your double cheese. Get your super-sized butt out of my seat!"

"You talk'n to me?"

"Yeah, Deniro. Move your carcass now."

Not later, not five years from now. Do it now. Put yourself on autopilot and just do it. It took me forever to get started because I believed 50 pounds was too big a wall to climb. However, it was the consistent choices every day that allowed me to get to minus 60 pounds. All of the sudden, minus 50 was there and past, and it took less than 6 months to get there. It wasn't like I climbed Everest, although I thought it would be like that. Why did I wait so long? Don't wait. Do not hate yourself, but hate what the years of neglect and lack of knowledge have led to. Commit yourself to change. Losing weight, even if it's 100 pounds, is definitely within the realm of human capability. You can do it; you are just making a bunch of fat cells get smaller. You are creating discipline and exerting control that you forgot you had. We can't control other people or external circumstances, but we can control ourselves. Let me repeat: we cannot control our external circumstances, but we can control our response to those circumstances. You can reach for a pint of Hagan-Daaz or that lovely Granny Smith apple—it's your choice. In the morning, your boss is still a jerk, your check is still late, the air conditioner in your mini-van is still shot, but you will at least feel a little better about yourself and the fact that you chose progress over self-destruction. Life is life; don't let it steamroll your health as well as your self-image. When you let go of this control, you have to learn to do two things. First, grab the reigns back quickly. Don't let a small slip turn into momentum for failure. Secondly, get over it! Get back on track and let yesterday be yesterday. So what if you're not perfect 100% of the time? Will 85 to 90% be better than where you are now? You bet it will!

AVERAGE JOE PHYSIOLOGY

Stress Eating is the Real Deal

You've heard the commercials for cortisol-reducing supplements. "Block the hormone that traps unwanted fat around your stomach..." I'm not sure if the supplements can do much to stop your adrenal glands from producing cortisol, but a valid point is raised. Many of us admittedly are "stress eaters" or "emotional eaters." There is a very good reason. Under stress, and your brain doesn't care if it's from being chased by a grizzly bear, deadlines at work, or watching the nightly news, your body goes into "fight of flight" response. Your heart rate increases, blood is shunted to your muscles for action, and stored carbohydrates (glycogen) are diverted from your liver and muscle into your bloodstream for the anticipated energy needs.

As the process slows – assuming you didn't get caught by the bear or your boss – that extra blood glucose gets stored as abdominal fat. It is directed mainly to your middle because only there can it be mobilized rapidly again for conversion to glucose. Your body is thinking ahead – for survival. The problem is we're getting more and more chronic daily stress and we're not using the released energy. It gets worse.

The storage of the new fat deposits signal the brain to shut off the stress response and the next phase of fight or flight is launched: operation refuel. The hard-wired expectancy of the nervous system is that after a stressful situation, energy will have to be replaced. Waves of cravings follow as part of the let-down from stress. Cortisol not only causes direct abdominal fat storage but intense carbohydrate cravings. (Just a side note: many researchers now directly link antidepressant drugs to obesity for this same reason. Apparently, we get locked into this step that involves bringing stress levels down when we take these medications.) Stress must be met head on with preparedness. When our daily lives create turmoil and intense hunger follows, you can combat it by relaxing, performing breathing exercises, walking away from the situation, drinking a glass of water, etc. This is to literally buy yourself time and direct your brain to de-escalate the situation. If you find yourself reaching for food, realize the situation at hand and make sure it doesn't lead to a binge. With this information you don't have to be dragged under the tow of this hormone; you can stay on top with planning.

Lone Ranger or Group Animal?

Some of this goes back to what I discussed above about internalization. It is okay to be by ourselves if we have obtained the information that we need. Being alone will allow us to get out and do what we need to do without having to wait on our friend or spouse to help us. However, we can be a good example to others and help them. My wife and her friend were great role models working out together and getting up early to exercise long before I ever realized that I could crawl out of bed with the chickens to walk on the treadmill. (Ever see a chicken walk on a treadmill? How do you think they get those plump, tasty drumsticks?) I never, ever thought I could get up before six to exercise, but guess what? I can.

Being with others can be a great motivator, but don't fall into the trap of allowing your gym time to be the social hour. It completely baffles me that in this world where every second is precious, people will go to the gym and in the middle of their workout stop and talk for a half an hour. I encourage people to form relationships, but do we really want to spend more time away from our families and sabotage our workouts at the same time? Partners can help push us, but they should never be a distraction.

As I discussed earlier, you are ultimately responsible for yourself, and you should never use your partner as an excuse for not doing what needs to be done. I'll give you another example. A patient and her friend have a signal that if one or the other is sick or too tired to get up at 5:00 a.m., they leave their porch light on. The other then is free to go to the gym and workout until they hook up again. This way there is never the excuse that "Oh, so and so didn't show up today, so I just slept in." You could fill in the blank for any excuse: "Oh, so and so brought doughnuts today and I couldn't offend them by not eating one." Uh, hello! Of course you can. Do something practical like staying out of the break room until it's actually time for lunch. Furthermore, if that person actually is offended and tries to make you feel guilty then ignore them. My wife has often said that she would much rather have me compliment her food rather than her looks. I have discovered, however, that I don't always have to eat two or three portions to prove that I love her. But that took a while for her to get used to. You are not a kid being extorted to eat every morsel. Many of us have to overcome our parents' and grandparents' Depression-era mentality that we have to clean our plate. Even more distressing is the number of us who dish out adult-sized portions to our children and then insist that they can't leave the table until they're finished. Kids often times have the inherent urge to stop eating so don't beat that out of them. Another example would be the child who after being told not to eat a cookie, runs up to you with a cookie in each hand saying, "Here, I brought you a cookie," eagerly anticipating that you will accept it and that he can happily munch the one in the other hand. We don't fall for that from our kids, so why should we fall for it from our coworkers? Who are we *really* cheating when we cheat?

It's the little daily choices we make that lead to big consequences. Your cells are replenishing and rebuilding every day, so how will you rebuild you? Will it be on the sand of sugar and the slippery slope of fat, or will it be on the rock of lean protein, healthy carbs, and small amounts of good fat? You don't have to get down to your goal in 90 days for some contest. It's not unusual to lose 20 to 30 pounds in 90 days, but what if it takes you 120 days? What if it takes two years? Don't give up. It's been 28 months for me and it seems like the blink of an eye. Two years will pass whether you are eating healthy or not. It may seem like a long time, but check back with me in two years. It'll seem like one day. You'll be loving life if you're leaner and fit.

The Fallacy of Control

Okay, I believe we need to pause here to clarify something. We want to help you regain control; we want you to have hope. With that in mind, you don't have to sit around and let life just happen to you or let it push you around. Thank God you are blessed with free will. Lower weight, blood sugar, blood pressure, and cholesterol are all important for better health. We want to try to get the out-of-control eating back to normal, so we provide a solid framework for guidance so you don't feel like you are alone wandering in the desert of diet misfortune. For those of you who are control-oriented, you have to loosen up a little and not crumble when you feel control over your nutrition slipping. We give you the flexibility so you don't have to be rigid with every single meal and snack.

If the addictive, destructive control of anorexia or bulimia is present then therapy is in order. Anorexia is far, far too complicated an illness to think that our "diet-obsessed" culture is simply to blame. People have been obsessed with appearance since the ancient Egyptians came up with cosmetics. Eating disorders have nothing to do with good mental or physical health or proper nutrition. Anorexics pathologically believe that by controlling what goes into their bodies they can control their anxiety, OCD, lives, or what others think of them. These harmful, distorted beliefs drive them to their destructive, and at times fatal, end. It is a devastating, incredibly hard illness to treat that often spirals out of control.

The disease process consumes entire families, and whatever can be done to combat this illness should be done. Saying "just eat more" doesn't begin to dignify the pain these families go through. Young people don't realize that anorexia can lead to death from heart failure or arrhythmias from electrolyte abnormalities. Even more disturbing is a trend we are seeing in adults who are under-eating or over-exercising in an effort to gain control of their lives. Ultimately the disease wins, and they and their families lose. If you or someone you know suffers from this illness, put down this book right away and seek help from a specialist trained in eating disorders. Often your family doctor or pediatrician is a good place to start, but they are not adequately versed in providing long-term follow-up care. The hardest step to take is realizing that you're not in control; anorexia is controlling you. If you have slipped near or past the edge of anorexia or bulimia, you have to reach out right now; you have to trust that you need help and that you have hope. Call your doctor right now.

Obesity can be just as devastating. Having a mother or father ripped from their family due to a heart attack, stroke, sleep apnea, or other problem can leave a family in ruin. Furthermore, it is my personal belief that far more people eat out of stress or feel out of control with over-eating than most of us realize. We believe that successful weight loss is about 80% nutrition and 20% exercise. You can lose all the weight you want with nutrition but still not be completely healthy. Exercise is very important.

The mentality of eating "whatever/whenever" leads to depression over doing something we know is self-destructive and self-defeating. Real control is enjoying doing what is right (within a flexible framework). Stop the out-of-control eating. There are too many land mines in convenience-foods in the form of added sugar and fat. It is there to keep you hooked. If you are running to five different practices for your kids or working two jobs, you are a target to be hooked for life. Take a couple of days to read this book, shop at the grocery, and implement a plan that will work for you. If you don't believe that you have time to prepare meals yourself, several companies are responding to the time constraints of our age with meals that have less sugar, are well-balanced, and contain plenty of vegetables. Sugar may make your mood better temporarily, but putting some sense of proper control back in your life will make you feel more confident and elevate your mood long-term. Trust me on this; I know first hand. Once you're on track with your eating, you will not want to go back to the same old same old. No one is a hopeless case. If I'm not, I darn well know you're not. Don't give up. We believe in you.

Eating Like a Youth

I love a certain part in the modern-day *Freaky Friday* where the Jamie Lee Curtis mind of the mother is trapped in the teenage body of her daughter played by Lindsay Lohan. (They're both so darned cute in that movie!) The mother's persona is savoring the french fries that she hasn't been able to have for years. She can get away with it now that she is in her daughter's high-metabolism, 17-year-old frame. Don't we wish sometimes that we could go back to that? We wish we could be able to "eat whatever we want and never get fat." (There's that "whatever/whenever" mentality.)

There are several problems with that reasoning. First of all, some teenagers start getting fat on that type of diet before they even get out of high school. We are teaching them incredibly poor nutrition that will carry into college and even early adulthood. Then the metabolism starts to slow down (although it is a very slow decline), we don't get as much exercise, and our abdomens continue to swell. It is much more the lack of movement as we age that is the culprit for the seemingly declining metabolism than an actual decrease in basal metabolic rate.

Furthermore, we think as adults that we ought to be able to put away a half a pizza and a six-pack (of soda, of course!) like we did in college and still be okay. We trick ourselves into thinking that if we down that kind of fare that "we are still young and vigorous without a care in the world." If we eat like that, we couldn't possibly be getting old or fat, even though we have to spend the night with a bottle of TUMS and Alka-Seltzer by our bedsides. Well guess what? We are getting older, there isn't a fountain of youth, Ponce de Leon was just an ancient version of Ashton Kuchar with a funny metal helmet, and we've all been *Punk'd*. Retro snacking (thanks *Thirtysomething*) and eating junk will make us feel briefly nostalgic, but it will simply accelerate our demise. Proper nutrition and exercise, although it is not nearly so much fun initially, are the only ways toward a healthy, vigorous life. Shooting hoops with your buddies and playing with the kids when you're 45 is a lot more fun than standing on the sidelines.

I believe that men sometimes have a delusion that mass equals health and dominance. "Hey, if I weigh 220 I must be the man!" All you are is bloated and sick. When I went on vacation (before I lost weight) I was in danger of being harpooned by Russian whaling ships if I strayed into the wrong waters. Being fit is being fit and there are no shortcuts. You'll look a lot more like the cover of *GQ* at a lean, mean 170 than a puffy 220.

What Would Mother Teresa Say?

Don't be afraid to throw left-over junk food in the trash. Isn't your health worth more than the half a bag of leftover chips that you *know* you will eat if you leave it in your cabinet after that party? Let's face it, there is absolutely no nutritional value to that type of food, so enjoy a little then pitch it. Why keep it around? For the kids? If you want to do something for your kids, then donate to St. Jude's or Jerry's Kids, but don't poison your children's little bodies with junk, and don't use that as an excuse to lead to the premature death of their parents. You don't have to be a human garbage disposal picking at pieces of your kid's leftovers on the way to the trash can. If you gave yourself too large of a portion, then save it for tomorrow or throw it away.

The Diet Docs' Rx, power spacing, and other structure provided in this book make it easier, but you will be faced with temptations of every kind. It doesn't have to be a big, dramatic deal, but you will have to choose to walk away from that piece of cake or from the dinner table some times. Planning ahead helps, but you can't prepare for everything other than the known fact that you need to face the food demons and walk away. Although it may be helpful in certain circumstances to have a support group to pat you on the back, you really don't need to have a pat for every little thing. Walk away simply because you choose to do the right thing. Then do it repeatedly.

Trick or Treat

We all have fond memories of getting treats as kids because that's exactly what they were—treats. We did not get them every day or even every other day. You may not want to eat your broccoli, Mr. Bush, but you need to. If not, you're still waking up with the same stress and problems in the morning, but now you may have diabetes and hypertension to contend with as well. If candy is in your house and it's too tempting, throw it away, walk out of the kitchen, or suck on a carrot stick. Just do whatever it takes to stay away from it during vulnerable times. Overeaters Anonymous has a great tip for this: HALT. When you decide to eat, are you really **H**ungry or just **A**ngry, **L**onely, or **T**ired? Before you start to put that bite in your mouth you need to ask if you are truly hungry or simply giving in to another emotion. Unfortunately for a lot of us men, that "L" stands for "lazy" when we don't want to spend the time to prepare proper food or dispose of junk that we don't need. Be practical. If you can't handle the bread basket at the table, then tell them not to bring it.

You may spend a lot of money on a meal out, but you won't throw away 10-cents-worth of half-eaten bologna? Think about it. You don't get a throwaway body. You have to take care of the one God gave you. Food is not an entitlement and good health is certainly not an entitlement either. Eating right is a sign of true maturity.

A Visit to the Vice Principal's Office: The Development of Discipline

Discipline is really the key. It is not a bad word, although many of us are convinced that it is. We are a fiercely independent nation and we don't want to be told we need to lose weight or exercise. Proverbs (5:23) tells us, "He will die for lack of discipline, led astray by his own great folly." You don't want to die do you? You can exercise as much choice as you want over your daily food intake as long as you're tracking within your personal Rx. But we must create healthy habits and stick to it. You will be shocked to see the discipline you have developed in the arena of nutrition carry over to other areas of your life. The development of healthy routines will lead to success.

You have to learn the power of the word "no" and give up the fallacy of control. You can develop discipline that creates habits which will allow you to withstand the curve balls life throws at you. You have been given "flexibility within a framework." These patterns allow you to get quickly back on track if you deviate. On a business trip? Say no to the high-fat, high-carb foods until you can find a good option. If you honestly cannot find anything healthy to eat—which

I believe happens very rarely—control the volume and get back on track with quality as soon as you can.

You know that there are vending machines in the airport, pop machines at the gas station, and fast food on every corner. There are no excuses, however, for showing up at the airport with an empty briefcase instead of one loaded with healthy alternatives.

The difference in a "cheat" meal and a "cheat" weekend is dramatic. You have to exercise discipline to say "no" to the idea: "Hey, I made it through the work week so let the party begin!" I see so many people who "diet" during the week then "eat normally" over the weekend. However, the weekend for them usually begins around noon on Friday and continues until Monday morning. Suddenly, they are "dieting" barely 50% of the time, and the "eating normal" (which usually is not "normal," but excessive) does not allow them to lose weight.

Even at the ball diamond on the weekend you can make good choices and have half a bottle of Gatorade, which may have a quarter of the carbs of a soda. Even better, get water. Take a protein bar with you. Eat a few peanuts, skip the cheeseburger, and eat when you get home. There are many options; it is your choice. It's not like someone kidnapped you and dropped you in the middle of the kindergarten t-ball game or soccer field with no warning and nothing to eat but burgers.

Make sure you have exercised the discipline of reading labels and food count books ahead of time to know what choices to make. The more time you have spent and the more knowledge you have stored in your brain, the easier it will be to make good choices and not be fooled. If it's true that you don't always need willpower, then you have to develop a plan ahead of time so you are not simply relying on being strong at the moment. Let's conclude this section as we started it, with a quote from the book of Proverbs: "Though it cost all you have, get understanding." Words to live by.

An Exercise in Adventure or Creature of Habit?

One of the things I believe about this program and staying consistent with your personal Rx is that whether you are adventurous or a person who likes ruts, you can do this diet. I believe that variety is important for good nutrition, but if you like having the same thing every day, either way can work in this plan. Make sure you take your daily multivitamin regardless just to make sure you're not creating deficiencies.

I really used this diet as an opportunity to try different meats, vegetables, and fruits that I haven't tried in years. Since I wasn't limited on what I could eat, as long as I stayed in my "range," I would try to find different things that appealed to me. Experimenting with protein shakes, bars, veggies, and dips made going to the grocery fun, especially for someone who doesn't cook very much. Taking cooking classes with my wife and learning about fish and ingredients (uh, they make other things out of tomatoes than just ketchup?) was wonderful. If you don't like this kind of stuff, then eat whatever works for you! But remember, fresh produce is an important part of any healthy diet. There is no way around that fact.

We sometimes have to do things we don't like to get healthy. (What do you mean you don't like spending 45 minutes on a machine that makes you feel more like a hamster on a wheel than a human?) I would love to walk around with one of those hats with a can of Mountain Dew on each side, a straw in my mouth, and a holster full of Pringles. But that won't get my blood pressure down or my lipids under control or make my joints hurt any less. Try different things until you find what works and lock in. Let's face it: do any of us really think that eating a half-pound cheeseburger without the bun is healthy? So you left out 25 grams of carbs so that you could get 55 to 60 grams of fat. Do you honestly think that was a healthy trade? Of course not.

I am a bit of a homebody, and as I settled into the middle months of the diet I found certain foods that I knew would help me everyday to stay on track. (I am so tempted to insert a shameless product plug here in hopes of getting cases of delicious and nutritious protein shakes so I could enjoy their chocolate goodness, but I would never do that.) Although that can lead to a little bit of boredom, it helped keep me focused, and I also found that I appreciated my splurge meals a lot more.

Layers of Protection

We have already discussed anorexia, but morbid obesity can also result from disordered thinking. One of the things that sadden me greatly during my practice of medicine is the person who packs on the weight as layers of protection against previous assaults. These assaults may have been sexual, physical, or verbal. These people believe that the extra weight offers layers of protection against unwanted sexual advances or makes them big and strong to stand up to a previous foe. The assailant from the past unfortunately continues to inflict damage on their victim. Please try to understand that if you are a victim of abuse or assault you can get therapy and begin to peel off the layers that threaten to destroy your physical health as well as your mental well-being.

Plan or Agenda?

Now that you are solidly focused on the goal of health, do you have a realistic plan or just simply an agenda? Is this book and your new-found enthusiasm for nutrition part of something that you want to incorporate for the rest of your life, or are you just trying to impress your wife? Is this just a way that you are trying to trick yourself into thinking that since you purchased this book that you are actually doing something about your weight? "I'm just going to go back to (fill in the blank with any previously-unsuccessful weight-loss program)." "My husband lost more than me. Men always lose easier then women." Blah, blah, blah. Don't buy "slimming" clothes, get slim! Get smaller sizes and give away your fat clothes. Read the book, make your plan, stick to it, and do not give up no matter what.

Of course, you are the only one who can do it. No one can force you. Feels good to have that much power doesn't it? No one can badger you into starting until you are good and ready. But if you are more than 20% above your ideal body weight, you are technically obese. And if you are 50% above your ideal body weight, you are morbidly obese. So I implore you, I beseech you (or any other Olde English verb you can think of): let's get going! That same power that keeps you prisoner can be turned into a power for good to free yourself. Remember, Peter Parker, with great power comes great responsibility. Don't eat like there's no tomorrow because if you do there may very well not be one. There are a whole lot of choices out there, so come on and make good ones.

CHAPTER NINE KEY POINTS

▶ 1) The statute of limitations on parental dietary misconduct is over – give yourself a break.

▶ 2) Time is on your side.

▶ 3) Have fun.

▶ 4) Don't rationalize. Let your weight-loss success be your reward.

▶ 5) Little daily choices lead to big results. Choose wisely, Grasshopper.

▶ 6) D-I-S-C-I-P-L-I-N-E isn't a 4-letter word; it's a 10-letter word. (That makes it 2.5 times more difficult, but don't fear it.)

▶ 7) If you have serious psychological issues regarding eating, do not hesitate to get long-term, professional help.

▶ 8) Have a plan, not an agenda.

▶ 9) You have hope.

CHAPTER TEN

PUTTING IT ALL TOGETHER

Come on, Doc, Does it Really Work?

You can take the most important step to ensure your success right now. When a client leaves my office for the first time, I can predict his or her success with indescribable accuracy. I observe people interacting with science and life. I see people succeed, and I see people fail. The best and most accurate information means nothing if you don't or can't apply it. My clients who take the initiative never fail. This first step is critical: it is simply to start now. Use the Six Week Program Guide (or your own notebook) and start recording your food intake *now*. Waiting until tomorrow will lead you to next week; next week will lead you to failure, and you may just throw away your last chance to gain total control over food, your health, and your physique. Start today. Sound like a broken record yet? (For you twenty-somethings, records are the prehistoric ancestors to discs.) Record everything you eat for a day or two as you make small changes that you easily recall from this book. Start fine-tuning your nutrition by making better-quality food choices, improving your meal spacing, concentrating on meal ratios, and reaching your target personal Diet Docs' Rx. Before you know it, you'll be feeling better than you thought possible, losing weight, and you'll be well on your way to becoming your own nutritionist.

Guaranteed?

It's hard for me not to guarantee success to everyone, because I know that success is *possible* if you follow the program. The greatest deterrent to your achievement once you get started is reaching too high a comfort level too soon. I occasionally have a client who starts with the incredible motivation that comes with the new understanding of nutrition. He or she starts losing two to three pounds a week, refers friends to our facility, and is overjoyed with the results. This client meticulously documents food and nutrient totals and consistently progresses. Then one day, progress slows; sometimes this person starts regaining weight. All of a sudden, either "it's just not working anymore" or they suddenly "have a slow metabolism." I ask to see their nutrition journal, and the reply is often, "Well, I quit writing things down last month." Translation: "I've lost my motivation. I'm cheating. In short, I'm no longer doing what needs to be done."

As soon as this client gets back on track—guess what? Their results pick right up where they left off. The point of this drawn-out example is that you must be consistent to reach your goal. It is so easy to slip upward into "maintenance" eating. You're still eating perhaps the right percentages of macronutrients, but add just a little too much food and the intake volume may take you out of the losing range and into the maintenance range. My advice would be to stick with your weight-loss level of food intake for as long as you can and then take a planned break where you increase your volume to a maintenance level to "catch your breath," regroup, and then go right back to progressing. I can't emphasize enough that your initial progress and understanding needs to be underlined by *consistency*.

Prepare to Win!

Once you've gotten off to a great start, prepare for a long journey of experimentation, changes, new understanding, and better integration of proper nutrition into your daily life. A shift in your thought processes regarding food has to occur. It is incredibly rewarding for me to see a client lose the 34th and 35th pounds, or to have a client reach the goal of losing 15 pounds in 8 weeks. However, I'm ecstatic when I see that client enjoying a higher quality of life a year later—without having gained any weight back. This long-term success has very little to do with me. I take great pleasure in knowing that clients took the right information and worked consistently hard to win what were perhaps great wars in their lives. I can educate and motivate, but ultimately it's you that will or will not succeed. We may all fall down once in awhile, but unfortunately not all of us will get back up. As the initial motivation wears off and the ice cream is no longer as easy to pass up, you have to remember who you're doing this for. You now have the tools to pick yourself up. You have a plan that's a proven success; you're no longer stumbling around in the dark. I know you can do it!

CHAPTER TEN KEY POINTS

▶ 1) Start right now!

▶ 2) Document meticulously.

▶ 3) Consistency, consistency, consistency.

▶ 4) It doesn't matter how many times you fall down, only how many times you get back up!

▶ 5) You're in this for life – be patient and enjoy the trip!

▶ 6) Prepare your mind for battle; prepare to win!!

CHAPTER ELEVEN

SIX WEEKS TO METABOLIC TRANSFORMATION

Let's Get Started!!

Many of my clients have attended a lecture or a one-on-one consultation with me and then received a copy of my previous book. I have seen a lot of "eureka" moments as clients start to understand past errors and connect the dots of sound nutrition. Rarely does a client leave without thinking they've found the missing link, excited to begin their new program. Rarely, however, do they start without getting overwhelmed by the sheer volume of new information. This six-week start is an incredible tool that will cement all the physiology you find on these pages into your eating habits—one step at a time! Following this six-week program has become as close to a 100% guarantee for your success as anything I have ever seen.

Week One

Week one has a single focus. We want you to get familiar with the charting system provided and begin the process of tracking your food intake. This week may be frustrating as you start measuring food, planning meals, and calculating nutrients for journaling. The rare person who fails often stops here. If you're committed to your goals, you'll survive this step and will have ensured your success. Take this week very seriously, and you'll understand why we feel it's the most critical. Once you go through the learning process of tracking your food, you'll have a literal databank of nutritional information memorized without even trying! As you look up foods, read nutrition fact panels, scour menus, and record your intake, you'll be amazed how easy it becomes.

At the end of the first week, you should be getting into your personal Rx ranges consistently. The first couple days will be hit and miss; don't expect yourself to be perfect. This week is a learning process to help you to understand the documentation and slowly get used to what those suggested protein, carbohydrate, and fat intake ranges mean in terms of real food. It's one thing to see numbers on paper and another to translate them into meals!

It may be a good idea to keep your personal Diet Docs' Rx card, which we provided at the front of the book, in your pocket or in your nutrition journal. Jot down the food counts for meals you frequently eat. That way you don't have to calculate them over and over and can make faster decisions on the spot.

At the end of this chapter, there is a sample daily food chart and a six-week "at-a-glance" spreadsheet. Record the all-important daily food, amounts, and times on a form similar to this. It will help you keep a running tally and in planning for the rest of the day. The weekly chart is a great tool to study trends and really zero in on what levels of food intake allow for different weight-loss paces. Without this objectivity, it's virtually impossible to learn and you may find yourself going nowhere fast.

Week One Steps to Success:

1) Record your beginning weight, body composition measurements (if you're having a professional monitor your body fat percentage), and your suggested nutrient intake totals.

2) Plan a sample day by creating meals that include quality foods as discussed in the book, meal volumes that are appropriate, meal times that fit in your schedule, and adjust the meal amounts until the total amount of protein, carbohydrates, and fat fall into your suggested ranges at the end of the day.

3) Plan ahead for the day and make sure you have the food available that you'll need.

4) Record food intake throughout the day.

5) Make adjustments for the next day if necessary; remember, this is the first week and you shouldn't be perfect yet!

6) At the end of the week weigh yourself. (Keep in mind that losing more than one to two pounds will initially be water loss.)

7) Review your week and focus on "lessons learned" so you can improve for next week.

8) Keep your Diet Docs' Rx card with you for quick reference.

Week Two

Hopefully you now agree that going through week one with diligence was critical to your success. Now you have a great base of experience to know what all those grams of protein, carbohydrates, and fat really mean in a day of food intake. Week two's objective is to refine your meals and work on making sure your program is going to be perfect for you, individually. Chapter three offered guidance in creating meals that would be fairly consistent in volume, timing, and quality so that your food will be properly consumed throughout the day. Recall that blood chemistry stability is a major factor in how you'll feel and how effective your weight loss will be. We want you to experience more energy than you thought possible and minimize your hunger. This is easily accomplished by focusing on the "nuts and bolts" of your food throughout the day.

First, this week will be a fair assessment of the amount of food you're consuming. The first week's weight loss was a combination of water loss and fat loss, but this week will allow a better look at actual fat loss. Two to three pounds for men and one to two pounds for women is about perfect. Faster loss may indicate that you're in danger of losing muscle, getting too hungry, and being prone to overeating. Review chapter two on how to adjust your nutrient numbers if you're losing too fast or too slowly.

Glance back through your first week's journal of your food intake. Check for the consistency of your daily numbers, spacing between meals, and meal volume. Are you too high or too low on protein, carbs, or fat? Were there some large gaps between meals (four hours or more)? We disagree with nutritionists who try to get people to have the exact same ratios and amounts of food at exact time intervals, but for all the reasons we discussed in chapter three, there has to be some consistency. The amount of flexibility we feel is appropriate is for your own hunger patterns and for schedule normalcy. It can be a scheduling issue as to when you can eat a whole-food meal and when you may need a protein bar or shake. These are elements for you to decide based on your social situation and based on your hunger, likes, and dislikes. If, however, you aren't seeing the results you want, you may have to revisit this step and make sure you're not sabotaging your progress out of convenience. We want to make things as easy as possible, but some foods may need to be sacrificed for you to progress.

Week Two Steps to Success:

1) Review your first week of journaling. Look at daily nutrient totals, meal spacing, and recall subjective thoughts such as hunger, energy level, and ease of meal consumption.

2) Alter your meal plans if necessary due to schedule inconvenience or hunger patterns. Experiment to see if you can improve for your own comfort level.

3) Purposely increase your variety of foods to expand your arsenal of potential meals and snacks.

4) Start journaling subjective comments so you can relate your body's response to what you're consuming.

5) Weigh yourself and determine if you're losing too fast or too slow. Adjust your program according to chapter two.

Week Three

Now you're over the hump and on your way to permanent success. Whether you realize it or not, you have altered your eating habits and have gained a great deal of invaluable knowledge by embracing this experience thus far. Those first two weeks constitute the largest "structural" steps in your program. You have fine-tuned your food volume for a typical day which will satisfy proper nutritional needs to lose body fat and maintain lean body mass. If you're losing too fast or too slow, keep adjusting your totals based on the information in chapter two. Excellent documentation of your nutrition is key to making sure you have as objective a guide as possible.

It's time to look at the details of the actual food you're consuming. This would be a good time to review chapter four and increase your understanding of carbohydrates. The amount of information can be a little overwhelming but success in this area will come from the details. When you're dieting, the glycemic index, carbohydrate volume per meal, and avoiding sugar and trigger foods becomes paramount. You want little rolling insulin fluctuations in your bloodstream, not mountainous spikes. The closer you stick to the physiological principles in these chapters, the easier it will be for you to succeed.

Carbohydrates, I must repeat, are the body's primary energy source. At this point in your program, you may feel some hunger return if you're generally not eating enough calories. Most people believe they are eating more food than normal just because of the increase in protein and fibrous carbohydrates and because power spacing helps them feel full. However, it's also a common pattern for people to start letting protein levels slide and start increasing carbohydrate intake again. If you are heading in this direction, it's a slow path back to a plateau. Keep your carbs in check because too much carbohydrate intake will block your body's need to use an alternative energy source—body fat.

Recall that blood chemistry stability is a great focus. Make sure you're not elevating carbohydrates too high at meals or leaving gaping holes in your day without enough. Look at your food journaling and make sure you have some balance in your meals and snacks. They don't have to be exact replicas of each other, but you should avoid major inconsistencies as you seek to end up within your carbohydrate range for the day. Too many in one meal and you'll end up lethargic and then very hungry. Too few for too many hours and you will also end up hungry and unable to pull in the reigns at the kitchen table.

Week Three Steps to Success:

1) Review chapter four regarding carbohydrates.

2) Review your daily nutrition intake and take steps to make sure it's consistent daily.

3) Use a good measure of balance in your carbohydrate intake meal to meal. Avoid too much in meals and avoid allowing too much time between meals.

4) Start paying close attention to the glycemic index and note which carb sources trigger hunger a short while after the meal and which ones delay hunger.

5) Weigh yourself and adjust your nutrient intake as described in chapter two if necessary.

Week Four

We like to view fat as a variable, second only to carbohydrates, that can be used to sustain body fat loss if manipulated correctly. Chapter five provides plenty of detail regarding the function of fat in the body and the differences between "good" and "bad" fat. The practical application of fat can be simplified. Once you have created some good habits, including the addition of some healthy unsaturated fats, you'll have to cut the saturated fats to a minimum to stay within your daily range. If fat intake is as moderate as we suggest and healthy fats are the dominant source, then dietary fat will never take the blame for lack of progress. However, if the table starts tilting toward an increased fat intake (especially with a higher inclusion of saturated fats), a cascade of events will take place. First, the calorie-rich fat may take you right up to a maintenance range of food intake from your planned calorie deficit. This is common in people who mistakenly think carbs are the only thing to worry about. A hefty handful of almonds may seem like the best thing to eat to avoid letting the carbs get too high, but if the extra fat increases the total calories for the day out of a deficit range, a day of fat loss is missed. Portion size and daily food volume are critical steps.

Second, fat can be absorbed straight from the bloodstream and into your fat cells. Too much fat in a meal on a day in which calories weren't low enough results in a lack of progress and may actually lead to regaining a small amount of fat. Excessive amounts of fat can only be used as energy successfully if carbs are near zero, such as in a ketogenic diet. As previously discussed, however, this isn't the best or easiest way to lose weight. Make sure you're not letting your dietary fat grams climb if you mistakenly tend to focus only on carbs.

The bottom line is to make sure you include a variety of healthy unsaturated fats wherever you can in your diet. Keep fat sources spaced evenly throughout the day. Spacing will make it easier to stay in your suggested totals, allowing for slower digestion and better maintenance of blood glucose levels. More importantly, it helps keep hunger in check.

Week Four Steps to Success:

1) Pick a variety of unsaturated fats that can be used as at least 50% of your fat intake.

2) Space fat intake as evenly as possible within meal structure.

3) Don't let fat intake creep up just to keep carbs down.

4) Perform your weekly review of nutrition journaling for consistency and check your body weight for progress. Make your best effort to correct problem areas in carrying out your program and adjust your program according to chapter two if necessary.

Week Five

Minimizing protein's role in weight loss would be a mistake. As a matter of fact, behaviorally it is one of the best indicators of a client's success. We won't repeat the body's utilization of amino acids for cell function (we don't want you to fall asleep and start drooling on your new Diet Doc book). We'll stick instead to what will help you lose and control weight permanently. Most who embark upon this journey will have to raise their protein to a level they're not used to. We certainly don't advocate an unsafe, unhealthy, or even unnecessary level of protein intake, but most of us just don't eat enough. That's a controversial statement since we can survive on very little, but we're after thriving, not surviving. Basal metabolic function requires approximately 50 to 70 grams of protein a day just to stay in "neutral," and that doesn't account for the potential increased needs to do the calorie deficit of dieting and exercise. So eat your protein!

When protein is consumed, it is digested slowly. Other foods eaten at the same time are therefore digested and absorbed slowly as well. After those meals, blood chemistry will be more stable for a longer period. Hunger will be lower and energy will be higher. You don't have to eat protein at every meal, but there are some key times. Breakfast is a good place to eat some protein to prevent hunger shortly thereafter. If you can't eat much protein at breakfast, make sure you get some in your first snack such as a protein bar or shake. Dinner is also a meal in which you want to have a whole-food protein source to help prevent late evening hunger. These suggestions are based on years of experience as to what can help you succeed, but should be coupled with your own personal observations of your hunger patterns and schedule preferences.

The practical side of protein that we mentioned in the first paragraph relates heavily to hunger. It may have taken you a week or two to get your protein levels up to your suggested ranges. While weight loss is steady and energy is increasing, it is easy to ride this high just because of the positive reinforcement. But eventually, the rigors of daily life start competing with that momentum and it's easier to make choices due to convenience instead of conviction. Protein intake starts decreasing, hunger therefore increases, and reflexively, carbohydrate consumption increases again. Voila: the recipe for slipping out of a body fat burning mode. I work with a lot of professional bodybuilders, and I have to tell you that what works for them will work for us. When fat has to come off, eating enough protein absolves hunger, creates a more fat-loss-friendly internal environment, and just pulls a lot of things into place. Scott and I have both discussed how we automatically lose weight faster when we include a protein shake or two as snacks. They keep blood sugar stable, cut cravings, and save more fat and carbs for meals. You can eat a whole-food protein source as a snack as well, but when you find it difficult to get enough protein, remember to choose habits that are easy to maintain.

Week Five Steps to Success:

1) Make sure protein levels aren't sliding downward.

2) Keep protein sources lean whenever possible. Save fattier selections for occasional meals.

3) Consider protein bars or shakes for snacks if protein levels are difficult to achieve.

4) Review your charting and look for a link between lower-protein days and increased hunger and possible increases in carb intake.

5) Unwanted hunger often is preceded by low-protein meals. Consider increasing protein at those meals.

6) Check body weight for progress and adjust nutrient numbers per chapter two if necessary.

Week Six

You're now coasting through the middle portion of your weight-loss program. Reviewing all the key points in this six-week program from time to time will help keep the driving principles in the forefront of your mind. You may also consider reading certain chapters again for additional assessment of your progress. Week 6 is dedicated to an evaluation of your progress and a management plan for the rest of your time in weight-loss mode which may be another 3, 6, or 18 months. After that, you'll arrive at the incredible day of being able to celebrate the success of reaching your goal and increasing your food toward maintenance levels!

Before we get there, however, let's keep our hands on the plow and make sure we have the good fortune of reaching that point. Look at your daily charting of protein, carbohydrate, and fat intake. Carefully compare that information to your weight-loss progress. Pay attention even to overall calorie intake. Calculate weekly averages for those statistics and look for the relationship between the level of food and macronutrients you're eating and your rate of weight loss. You should be able to see a causal relationship between the two. You can observe with clarity and precision how much food you can eat each day (on average) and lose one pound, two pounds, or whatever your healthy desired rate, based on these records. Now you may see one reason we dictate that this documentation is key to your success. You have created a database that will enable you to manage your weight control for as long as you wish.

That is exactly our goal for the remainder of your program. Decide what pace you would like to continue (based on our recommendations of safe weight loss and your own comfort level), and plan meals and daily nutritional totals accordingly. Keep monitoring your progress and recording your food intake as you add to your knowledge. Understand that there will be an occasional setback or a social situation at which you anticipate not "eating perfectly" according to your plan, but if these are infrequent, you'll see your progress continue.

Week Six Steps to Success:

1) Review weekly weight-loss rate and compare with weekly averages of all three macronutrients.

2) Compare the relationship of this data for accurate estimations of the food intake required for different rates of weekly weight loss.

3) Celebrate the completion of your first six weeks!! (Yahoooooooo!)

NUTRITION JOURNAL

DATE: _____ WEEK: _____ DAY: _____ WEIGHT: _____

MEAL	PORTION SIZE	FOOD CONSUMED	TOTAL GRAMS PER MEAL			CALORIES
			Pro	Carb	Fat	
1						
2						
3						
4						
5						
6						
7						
		TOTALS FOR DAY				

Monthly Nutrition Log

Week One

Day	Protein	Carbs	Fat	Calories	Comments	Weight
1						
2						
3						
4						
5						
6						
7						
Averages						

Week Two

Day	Protein	Carbs	Fat	Calories	Comments	Weight
1						
2						
3						
4						
5						
6						
7						
Averages						

Week Three

Day	Protein	Carbs	Fat	Calories	Comments	Weight
1						
2						
3						
4						
5						
6						
7						
Averages						

Monthly Nutrition Log

Week Four

Day	Protein	Carbs	Fat	Calories	Comments	Weight
1						
2						
3						
4						
5						
6						
7						
Averages						

Week Five

Day	Protein	Carbs	Fat	Calories	Comments	Weight
1						
2						
3						
4						
5						
6						
7						
Averages						

Week Six

Day	Protein	Carbs	Fat	Calories	Comments	Weight
1						
2						
3						
4						
5						
6						
7						
Averages						

CHAPTER TWELVE

PITFALLS AND OBSTACLES

Remember the old video game *Pitfall?* Sometimes when you are navigating through a diet plan you feel like you are swinging on vines over the gaping mouths of the alligators. Dieting has its pitfalls and obstacles. We have dealt with the ones that occur in the realm of emotion and psyche in an earlier chapter. Now let's face some of the things we have seen time and again that may grab you by the leg and put your diet into a death spiral. This is by no means the only list, and we would love to hear from you to add to these contents! We provide this chapter to be supportive and to let you know that others have gone through some of the same things you have. There will be practical tips as well to help you cope with these dietary "danger zones."

Some of these areas may seem quite obvious and others may be like quicksand. Even after you fall into one of these traps you may be left slapping your head and asking yourself, "How could I have done that? How could I have been so stupid?" Don't worry. We have all been there at one time or another. Your best defense against these types of problems is to make like a Boy Scout and be prepared. As we discussed in the psych chapter, you will face temptations, so plan ahead how you will handle them. Also, keep yourself well-supplied with good foods that are easy to take along. Even better, arm yourself with the knowledge contained in these pages and you can make good choices no matter where you are. Remember in the first Indiana Jones movie, *Raiders of the Lost Ark?* (You know, the good one; not the one where he is sitting around with the future Mrs. Spielberg eating monkey brains.) Picture that great fight scene in the market. We want you to be like Indiana Jones with a holster full of dietary knowledge and your diet foes to be like the big dude with the sword. You get the picture. (I wonder if any of the food count websites list the protein content for monkey brains?)

Time is on Your Side

Or is it? Too many of us live as if we don't have a microsecond to spend on ourselves. We already talked about the excuse of being too busy. Some people frankly are unbelievably busy. However, we always make time for what is important. Make time for this. Check your cabinets and see how much healthy food you have right now. If you are well-stocked then simply allow a little more time at the store as you ponder a variety of healthy choices. If you don't have much at home, make a trip to the market now. Not later; now. Strike while the iron is hot! Take that enthusiasm that you have for the diet and use it to your advantage. Procrastination only will lead to more excuses. Also, remove any food that may be a potential obstacle. I would recommend periodically cleaning out any unhealthy foods that have accumulated from parties, restaurants, or the like. Some professionals will encourage you to put "the kids'" junk food in an out-of-the-way place to make it harder to get. I don't recommend that for several reasons. First of all, the first few weeks of the diet are crucial, so the kids and your spouse may just have to live a little sugar-deprived for that time. Second, you will hopefully be trying to get your kids to eat healthy as well. The only thing you are "depriving" them of is an early start on obesity, diabetes, and heart disease. Finally, you *know* where the "junk drawer" is unless you've watched *50 First Dates* one too many times. I have been known to repel from the ceiling like Tom Cruise in *Mission Impossible* to try to get that last Hershey Kiss my wife has hidden in the top of the closet. Although it was fun trying to outsmart her, it was ultimately a game. If I wanted to be serious, I had to stop playing those kinds of games. Let's face it—I couldn't outwit her anyway. I know the junk is there; I also know I can grab anything I want at the gas station. Develop the discipline of avoidance.

Preparation really is a key. True, it takes more time to clean a bunch of grapes than pop open a box of crackers or a bag of chips, but clean the grapes ahead of time and store them in the refrigerator. Then you can throw a few in your mouth when you are hungry. Nature's pre-packaging of grapes, berries, and apples makes for a very quick snack. Fruit does have carbs, but let's face it, any diet that makes you believe that fruit is not healthy is a joke. Too many carbs are bad for you, but the few carbs in a handful of blueberries are nothing in comparison to white bread or a potato. Also, fruit is high in antioxidants and fiber. Bodybuilders and people who are health conscious will often grill many chicken breasts ahead of time so that they can quickly warm one in the microwave and have a meal. You may not feel like cooking in advance, but it will help you save time later when you really need it.

Buy in bulk once you know what you like. I'm not talking about buying the 50-gallon drum that you know will go bad after you only use a third of it. We're talking about buying two or three weeks of shakes, bars, frozen meals—whatever will be some of your mainstays—so you won't run out of ammunition.

Another key is being patient. We cannot emphasize enough that you are developing a lifetime of eating and exercise habits so don't expect to look like a cover model in a few weeks (unless you're Cindy Crawford already—Cindy, I told you I'd autograph a copy for you, you didn't have to buy this at the bookstore). That is completely unrealistic. True results only come with time. Learn a little more each week. Many people believe that it takes anywhere from one to two months to really get "dialed in" on the nutritional and exercise points. After a few weeks you should feel very confident about what your body can do and the ensuing months will "toughen" you up as you settle in for the long haul. You will also be able to see how you can enjoy certain foods without them leading to a disaster unless they are a "trigger food" which brings us to our next point.

Trigger Happy

Is there anyone out there who doesn't have a trigger food? Anyone? You in the back row? Trigger foods are foods that if you start, you will have a terrible time stopping. To borrow a famous phrase, "No one can eat just one." Don't mess with fire and don't tempt fate. (Maybe we should call this the pitfalls, obstacles, and cliché chapter.) We have seen people with amazing will power who can eat a few bites of cake or chocolate, but we believe those people are few and far between. If there are certain trigger foods on which you know you will gorge, then just avoid them, especially during the first several weeks of your diet. Even during your weekly "splurge meal" learn to start practicing moderation with these foods. Later, as you enter maintenance, you will have learned to manage those foods without sabotaging yourself.

Trigger foods often are full of carbs that will cause huge insulin spikes. You will then want to eat more and more, and you may find your cravings that had vanished during your months of healthy eating return with a vengeance. This is a bit of the fallacy of very low-carb diets—we are never really cured of our "carb addictions." Carbs release brain chemicals that make us feel good. We want them. The best we can hope for is to control them over time. As we have said, if we let carbs get too low, our brains don't work well and we get grouchy. (Just ask Joe's wife when he's dieting for the Mr. International contest. Tracy has threatened to send him to live with us more than once during those times.) If we eat too few carbs over an extended period of time, important hormones get low, our metabolism falls, and we don't feel well. It is indeed critical to eat the proper amount of carbs to avoid the previous pitfalls.

Oh, Those Pesky Hormones

Lower levels of carbs over an extended period of time can lead to decreased testosterone and thyroid hormone. I definitely had a time with this when I dropped my carbs below what Joe recommended. These decreases in hormones can lead to feeling somewhat depressed. The way to combat that problem is first to eat the recommended carbs in your personal Rx! Second is to increase your carbs incrementally, as discussed in chapter two, if you're losing too quickly. Finally, you can try something called "cycling." The Tour de Klemczewski. (Try to say that three times fast.) If you develop feelings of lethargy, which do not appear in all clients, you can increase your carbs slightly one or two days a week until that feeling passes. You may need to persist with that for a month or two until you get back on track. It is important you get these hormones back on line because you have to have the right frame of mind to be able to persist with a healthy eating plan over time. Let's say for example that your carb intake should be 70 to 90 grams per day. You know you have the splurge meal on the weekend, so a good strategy to avoid feeling too carb depleted during the week would be to stay close to 70 grams for 2 to 3 days, then up to 90 grams for a day. If you still feel symptoms of having carbs too low (weak, fatigued, shaky, or lethargic) make sure your protein and fat is up to the max level. Secondly, change carb sources around a bit. Despite even the glycemic index, some people just do better on some carbs versus others.

Plateaus—I Give Up!

"I didn't lose enough; I give up!" How many of us have said that at one time or another while dieting? Embrace the concept of delayed gratification. First of all, don't give up. Second, problem-solve. If you haven't lost enough, why is that? Have you not been documenting, watching your portion size, or reading your labels? Also, if you gained, it may not have been from exactly what you ate the day before, but perhaps several days ago, especially if it was high-fat. Sodium status may have affected your weight. (Did you pay a little visit to the Chinese restaurant?) So many things may affect your weight. Again, do not give up. If you are losing one to two pounds a week, you are doing great! You may lose at a much faster clip initially, but most people eventually settle into a healthy and sustainable one to two pounds per week pace. That is a perfect rate to keep weight off permanently. Also, what is your new "set point?" Isn't it easier to stay at 140 now instead of hovering at 150? I bet that it is. You may simply not need to weigh yourself as often if it brings your mood down. It's okay to vent a little, but what's the alternative—going back to the same lousy habits? Stay on target.

Plateaus during weight loss are not unusual. During my six months of intense weight loss, I experienced two plateaus. One lasted three weeks and one lasted four weeks. This slowing of weight loss can be very frustrating, but often that phase will end with a big loss of pounds. As the days mount up during a plateau and there is no loss on the scale, the temptation will be to give up and look in the mirror and say, "See, I told you so. I can't do this. Why did I think that I could ever succeed?" I have been right there with you. Exercise the discipline and stay the course when you know you're being precise with your personal Diet Docs' Rx, power spacing, and food quality. If you're not, it's not a plateau—it's a problem. Be honest with yourself and correct it. Do not give up now, or it is simply a self-fulfilling prophecy. Joe would tell me, "Just stick with it. Stick with it." I felt like the guy in *Star Wars* flying down the trench in the Death Star with his commander telling him, "Stay on target, stay on target!" only to get barbecued by Darth Vader. I even thought about telling Joe where to "stick with it," but I believed in the program. I couldn't argue with my success so far and the success of others I had observed. Lo and behold I did break through the plateaus and reached my goal. Hey, he was right! Well, duh! He's only helped thousands of people lose thousands of pounds in his career.

The reason you will smash through a plateau is because of the principles that we have discussed in the earlier chapters. You are eating below the maintenance level of calories for your size so your body has no choice but to eventually relinquish some of your fat as fuel. Your fat cells are not like the shark in *Jaws*, stalking you and just waiting for you to mess up. It is a biochemical reaction and those little suckers won't have any choice but to shrink!

Mommy, I'm Bored!

You know what? Sometimes nutritious food and exercise are boring. There, I said it. Time to revoke my diet guru card. Going to work every day can be boring, going to school can be boring . . . but you know what? Good health is never boring. Running with the kids for more than a minute isn't boring, playing tennis with your wife isn't boring (exasperating but never boring), hiking outside enjoying the world isn't boring, and living to see your great-grandchildren definitely isn't boring. Nutrition and exercise are the vehicles to get us there. Variety is the spice of life—or is it the staff of life? No that's bread, but I know that the mention of the word "bread" in any recent diet books may lead to immediate pelting of my house with cans of protein shakes.

Take a vacation from strict dieting for a week. Just increase your carbs daily by 25 to 50 grams, but still with healthy food. If you must take a rebellious total vacation from dieting, notice how you feel when you start back eating poorly. Use that feeling to help stoke the desire to stay on track. Cross training is certainly a good thing when it comes to exercise, and the same can be applied to eating. I really believe that although most of us are creatures of habit, if you have wholeheartedly embarked on this journey of nutrition, you won't tire of learning new things. Consequently, just keep on looking for new options to fuel your body. Do the same with exercise. Tired of walking on the treadmill? Get on the bike or the elliptical machine or take a kickboxing class. Tired of walking outside? Get an indoor exercise video to use during the winter months. Exercise and nutrition are not a burden; they are an incredible gift and blessing. Rekindle the desire to work through the inevitable patches of boredom that may strike. Take a break, but do not take a permanent vacation. Set new goals for your weight, exercise, or nutrition. Challenge yourself to stay motivated and fresh. Run with a friend in the local Race for a Cure or walk for March of Dimes. You can do it.

I'm Too Old and I'm Falling Apart!

This may be one of the most legitimate pitfalls. Multiple problems such as antidepressants, arthritis, sleep apnea, thyroid disease, heart medications, female hormone replacement, and diabetes all can lead to weight gain or difficulty in losing. Don't let that defeat you. I have definitely seen many diabetics and patients on thyroid medication who have lost weight with this diet. Losing weight will help decrease back and arthritis pain and will make diabetes and hypertension easier to control. Medication may make it harder to lose weight, but if you are still alive, your metabolism is still working, although its performance may not be optimal. Don't use medications or medical conditions as an excuse to quit working on nutrition and exercise. Realize that it may take longer to reach your goals, and you may have to modify your exercise program to fit your medical condition. Once you are aware of your medication's side effects, you can work within the framework that the medication allows. If you're not making progress, you can discuss with your physician if there is an alternative with fewer side effects. I would also caution you, however, to not use diet and exercise as an excuse to come off your medication too soon. Many people don't want to take medication, and if you can use nutrition and exercise to discontinue your diabetes, hypertension, or cholesterol meds, that's great and is obviously one of our goals. But don't *even* think about doing that unless you have been closely monitored by and in discussion with your physician.

Medications may simply make us hungrier; but now we have the information to make good choices instead of high-fat or high-carb foods. "Comfort foods" don't give us a lot of comfort as our bellies are pushing the rivets on our jeans to their maximum stress point. I have even seen people even in their mid-70's lose weight, especially to help decrease stress on their bodies prior to surgery. It can be done no matter what the age with the proper supervision.

The Social Dieting Nightmare

How can I tell Aunt Ella that I don't really want another slice of her sausage and beef pie with the cheese crust? Situations like this are guaranteed on vacation and even at work. You'll succeed a lot faster when you get the "Oh, what the heck, one won't hurt me" mentality out of the way. Family, unfortunately, is often the worst about using that form of guilt. You wouldn't walk up to an alcoholic and say, "Oh, you've done so well the last few weeks. Here, have a drink." Avoid the habit of feeling obligated. You have to decide. Talk to your family members in advance and let them know that you don't want to hurt their feelings, but you are trying to lose weight. (Tell them you're on a healthy eating program, tell them you've been recruited by The Diet Docs . . . do whatever it takes.) Don't let them sabotage you with guilt. Smile politely and move on. The same goes for coworkers. It is hard when someone brings in a treat and everyone is telling you how great it is. It is hard to walk away, but just plan to do it. In our little office of 15, there always seems to be a birthday, retirement, or special occasion. In a bigger office it could be even worse. Until you get yourself completely locked in, the polite but firm "No" will be your greatest weapon.

When Will the Pain Stop?

As I sat massaging my wife's feet after a particularly hard cardio class, she moaned, "Scott, when will the pain stop?" Being the thoughtful, caring husband that I am, I quickly replied, "Never!" Your muscles will be sore and you may develop trigger points that will benefit greatly from physical therapy or massage therapy. As you get stronger and your muscles become accustomed to actually being used, the soreness will become less and less. You need to consult your physician to determine when things are serious, and as we discussed earlier in the book, you should have a complete physical and comprehensive discussion with your physician before beginning any exercise program. For my wife, orthotics (to help her feet) allowed her to progress to running and an even higher level of fitness. I personally stayed away from physical therapy because I thought it would take too long, or that it wouldn't really work all that well for me, even though I've sent thousands of patients for therapy. (Sorry all you therapists out there; that was my own ignorance.) However, after having a shoulder that only worked at 50% capacity for years, I finally submitted to therapy once or twice a week for a few months along with some chiropractic, and now my shoulder feels the best it has felt in 15 years.

L'Oreal Syndrome

"Because after all, I'm worth it." Watch out! Overindulging after success can spin you back to failure. Maybe movie stars are worth it, but if they overindulge they can have a fleet of plastic surgeons fix whatever they desire. It may not hurt to reward yourself in a regimented fashion, but be very careful; it was that sense of entitlement with food that led to the overindulging in the first place. A moderate splurge meal once a week will give you something to look forward to and will allow you to still maintain your discipline.

Work-at-Home Moms/ Corporate Moms

Both our wives are work-at-home moms. Joe's wife, however, has the benefit of living with someone who really knows what he is doing and has made fitness a lifelong commitment. My wife has the burden of living with a slacker. She actually gave me a lot of advice on this portion. Work-at-home moms face multiple problems: convenience, constant access to food, lack of time to exercise, and boredom. Funny, moms at the office face those same problems! Convenience is a problem that all of us face whether it's stopping by the drive-through on the way home after gymnastics or giving a Pop Tart to the kids for breakfast as we are trying to get the oldest out the door and go over the middle child's spelling words. This is where shopping and prep time are very important. Make a double batch of a healthy entrée and freeze half of it. (Don't let it sit out and eat it!) Buy some low-fat peanut butter, berries, low-carb/low-fat yogurt. Change your kids' and your own eating habits. It only takes five minutes to eat a bowl of high-fiber cereal (trust me, I've timed it), so get up five minutes earlier and skip the doughnut at the office. Your health and your children's health are definitely worth the five minutes.

Moms face the problem of what my wife calls "the grazer mentality." Since she is in the kitchen a large percentage of the day—preparing meals, cleaning up, working on projects at the kitchen table with the little ones—she is constantly tempted to munch and she only has to walk a few feet to have something. At work, there may be a constant supply of Krispy Kremes in the break room, reps with gift baskets, or a candy machine that's right on the way to the rest room. That bag of M&M's in the desk drawer will unfortunately sometimes work better than a Valium.

If you find yourself glancing at the clock and feeling hungry, you will know that you will have a meal or a healthy snack coming up. You don't need to grab the junk. Don't nibble off your kid's plates (you wouldn't nibble off a coworker's plate would you? If you do, we really need to talk). You may need to change a few of your habits such as playing board games in the living room instead of the kitchen. It is just as easy to keep dried fruit, nuts, or protein nuggets in your desk as that bag of candy that will leave you tired and run down.

Keep the fridge and the cupboards stocked with healthy food, get rid of the junk food drawer, and then there's nothing there to tempt you or your kids. Remember that you are teaching them a lifetime of healthy eating, and you are not depriving them of anything. We spend a lot of time teaching them about values, sports, school, and life and we cannot neglect their health as well. Obviously it has to be age-appropriate, but we teach them that there are choices to be made in life about drinking, drugs, and smoking, so why shouldn't we educate them about choices of food? I believe one reason is that we're afraid we'll create eating disorders in our children when we emphasize diet so we ignore it. We also like to see our kids happy and what lights them up more than candy or dessert?! Of course, another reason is our hypocrisy. It's a lot harder to teach your kids about nutrition with chocolate chips wedged between your teeth. Actually there are great ways to work with your kids on nutrition and we are working on very practical solutions, but this book is about you. Your example, good or bad, is the most important impression you'll make on your children. My girls actually came up to me and patted my stomach saying they were glad I wasn't their "fat" daddy anymore. My son would talk to me as I ran on the treadmill and then he would actually hop on it when I was done. We are by no means perfect and are still working toward our goals, but I cringe to think where my family would be if we hadn't started.

My Spouse isn't on Board

This is a big problem. As anyone can attest who has tried to quit smoking when their spouse is still puffing away, it is very difficult. Trying to diet when your soulmate is sitting there eating cookies and ice cream after dinner and saying, "Mmm, mmm, good," is just plain hard! Some spouses will actively try to sabotage you because they are insecure about the way they feel. They may believe that they cannot have the same kind of success that you are experiencing. They may fear that if you get in shape, you will be a little too attractive to the opposite sex. Another problem may simply be that they really don't want to have anyone telling them what to do.

The bottom line is this: you are an adult and no one can control what goes in your mouth but you. No one should try to sabotage your health, especially if they claim to love you. There will need to be some frank discussion about some of these issues if you run into resistance. Notice I say discussion and not fight. Reassure your sweetie that you want to be with them a long time and that is why you are trying to take care of yourself. Have the quiet confidence to eat right. Lead by example and respect the fact that your husband/wife may not be at the same point in their life as you. That is okay—respect the difference. You cannot badger your spouse into dieting; it must come from them.

My wife exercised for several years before I firmly got with the program. Any of her badgering launched me into an immature binge of getting a double scoop of Rocky Road and an "I'll show you" mentality. Over time, I realized simply that she loved me and wanted to keep me around (and not just for my life insurance).

Rebel without a Clue

That nasty state of rebellion can derail any diet plan (with sincere apologies to Mr. Tom Petty and his Heartbreakers). No one wants to be told what to do.

You have to be honest with what you want out of life. If you are reading this, I honestly believe that you want to be leaner, healthier, and to feel better. You don't need to waste time with the notion of, "Who the heck do these guys think they are?" Maybe every once in a while it's okay to ask that. Then if you want to have one of those days—or even weeks—go right ahead. Notice how your intestines behave, what your energy level is like, what happens to your mental clarity, and what the scale does. If you have slid back into poor eating habits, I believe you will find that all of your systems do not function nearly as well. Then you will remember why you decided to start eating in a healthy fashion in the first place. Use that independent streak to your advantage to get and stay healthy. Maybe you can change that "Born to Eat" tattoo to "Born to Eat Right."

Stress/Mood Eating

This is one of the most difficult pitfalls to avoid. The first step in avoidance is preparation. Preparation against this problem comes in two forms. The first is by having plenty of healthy foods around so if you binge a little, you won't do too much damage. The second is to realize that you will binge eat due to stress at some point. Some people are fortunate enough to not eat (which is a problem unto itself) when they are stressed rather than finding solace in food. However, many have found comfort in chocolate or other things—that's why they call it "comfort food." There may be times when the stress eating starts, and we don't even realize it. We may be half way through a pint of Hagan Daaz before we even know what hit us! As soon as you recognize you're eating due to stress, stop! You may be able to salvage the day and get back on track. You may go over just a bit, but not lose your progress for the entire week. The only serious "damage" will be if you keep going.

Recall the Average Joe Physiology section from chapter nine regarding the hormone cortisol. Use the HALT method and think why you are doing what you are doing. Sometimes you may have to have a stare down with your food and know that you can walk away from that doughnut that's taunting you.

If stress eating is too much a part of your life, deal with the issue; don't hurt yourself. Don't underestimate counseling if necessary. Now you are starting to develop the healthy mental discipline as well as physical discipline. Keep it up. Just as diet and exercise go hand in hand, so do the mental and physical portions of proper nutrition.

The Burden of Keeping It Off

If you are uncomfortable with compliments and the new-found attention you will get from your weight loss, keeping the weight off may be difficult. I can hear a collective "Whatchu talk'n 'bout, Willis?" coming from our readers. I mean, isn't this what all of us are striving for? Yes, but if you are on the shy side and people are showering you with compliments, it may seem easier at times to retreat back into the shell of protection provided by the extra weight. The weight sometimes would allow you to "fly under the radar," which you may be more comfortable with.

There's another related danger that can be quite serious. If I'm at a function and a patient who I've worked with on weight loss sees me, they always bring up food. "I'm not eating that, Dr. Uloth, don't worry." "Oh, Dr. Uloth's here, now I can't even eat that cookie I was going to have." And I feel the same pressure! How can I be a good example if I publicly eat a brownie?! We advocate the splurge meal for physical and mental reasons and we're big fans of flexibility that would allow a little "junk" food at occasions like this if it still fits in your daily food volume goals. But because of this pressure of being seen "eating something bad," it can force us to be closet eaters. Bad news. Don't do it. Joe jokingly loves to eat junk in front of clients just to prove this point: in moderation, especially once you've reached your goals, a *small* variety of "non-health" food is normal and fun.

Success can even become a pride issue. I tended to let people focus on "my achievement" rather than giving credit to Joe, my wife, and my commander-in-chief, God. I needed to take the focus off of me and back on the fact that this project is about health and not just a certain look.

I remember wishing I were a year down the road so that all my patients would have seen "the new me" and I could finally stop talking about it! I began to believe that maybe it would be a little easier if I gained a little bit of the weight back so that people wouldn't focus on it so much. However, I knew my health would suffer. You are the same person inside.

I've Blown It

So I just might as well give up. This is a tremendous dieting pitfall. Two things happen with this type of thought pattern. We either slip into a state of self-defeating behavior where we continue to eat and eat because we can't believe that we could ever succeed in the first place. We might use it as an excuse to indulge. "Well, if I've already blown it I might as well keep eating." When you're in a moderate calorie deficit and you start eating simple carbs, it's hard to stop. Your body will want more.

Psychologically, most of us will contribute to the backslide with thoughts like, "I might as well finish this off and get it out of my house," or "I've been so good that this really won't set me back and I'll start again tomorrow." Some people mistakenly think that their body won't absorb much carbohydrate if they saturate themselves. Certainly your body can't use *all* those carbs, but it *will* absorb them and turn them into triglycerides to be stored as fat. Remember, your body doesn't know the difference; it is simply built for survival. Your brain is the computer that better tell your mouth when to stop! It can happen way too fast. You have to have a well-rehearsed emergency response plan to avoid a binge such as drinking a big glass of water, giving yourself a quick pep-talk, and getting away from food. Surrender is not an option.

Too Much of a Good Thing

Nothing is free. Even protein has calories! It is important to remain in your personal Rx. Each of the macronutrients have a purpose in the body. What makes most fad diets harmful or ineffective is that they eliminate one or two of the macronutrients or make one or two of them an unlimited option. As we already mentioned, this is for marketing purposes; you have to be unique to have a bestseller, right?

There are minimums and maximums to protein, carbohydrates, and fat if you want to walk that fine line of consistent weight loss with no harmful effects. If you eat too much protein your body can convert it to glucose, negating the need to utilize body fat. When total calories are too high at a meal, protein can even be converted into body fat. Make sure to read your labels and watch portion size. It's all about balance.

The Anatomy of Failure

Did you ever wish that you had J. Lo's backside or Nicole Kidman's shoulders? How about Brad Pitt's abs? While it is great to have goals, some people may focus on one body part so much that they ignore the progress that they have made. They may either turn to things such as plastic surgery or use that inability to look a certain way as an excuse to give up. We are all under certain anatomical restraints and we should try to maximize our potential rather than focusing on the one problem area. I once watched a reality TV show that presented the story of a young man that had a great physique but had plastic surgery to have calf implants! He thought his calves didn't look very good. How often do you really look at a guy's calves? He was willing to risk infection, scarring, or potentially even death to make his calves bigger.

When is enough enough? If you are healthy and lean, you will naturally look great! I know that "healthy" isn't always the greatest motivator until you're facing severe medical problems, but don't wait that long. Have you lost weight? Is your blood pressure down? Is your hear rate lower? Are your lipids better? Are you more energetic? Is your waist size down? Are people complimenting you? The list could go on and on. Realize the big picture and enjoy the process.

This is where smaller goals can help. If you have to lose 100 pounds and it has taken 9 months to lose 50, it may be easy for you to throw your hands up, wondering if you'll ever make it. But, you've lost 50 pounds!! Celebrate meeting your monthly goals, look at every 10 pounds as monumental.

But Dr. Atkins Will Let Me Eat . . .

Some diets talk about pasta, pizza, and beer. Others talk about plenty of eggs, cheese, and meats. Isn't that really the problem? Does the medical community seriously want to propagate "epidemic, life-threatening conditions?" You don't have to count calories? Well of course you do! It's just a matter of how you do it and how you manipulate those calories to make it easier to decrease your hunger and maintain your metabolism. But what if I don't like some foods? Find something healthy that you do like. It doesn't have to be like an episode of *Fear Factor*! Don't think you can eat a lot of high-fat food or uncounted carbs and be healthy or reach your goal.

Isn't Exercise Enough?

This is one of the difficulties I ran into after I had actually lost all my weight and was in maintenance phase. It transpired about 10 months into the program around the time of multiple birthday parties (mine, my wife's, and my daughter's) and holidays (Halloween, Thanksgiving, and Christmas). I couldn't forgo all those treats, and let's face it, what's better than a fun-size Snicker's pilfered from the trick-or-treat bag? I believed that since I was now exercising regularly that I could have a little dietary indiscretion and "get away with it." Of course a little turned into a lot and before I knew it I had gained about 8 to 10 pounds back! I kept saying that I would "hit it hard" again after the first of the year, but with two weeks to go until New Years, I realized I had better get back on the wagon quickly before I had gained 15 to 20 pounds.

Exercise is a cornerstone to any diet/physical fitness program, but exercise is not sufficient if you are eating loads of high-fat, high-carb foods. Exercise will give you more freedom to enjoy yourself once in a while. It will give you the confidence of knowing that you are in good shape and feel invigorated. However, exercise alone is not enough. The problem is that too many calories are shoved into small convenient packages such as soda, chips, and candy that can stuff us with 600 to 700 calories in a matter of minutes yet we don't feel full.

Don't go long stretches simply trying to rely on exercise. Diet and exercise must go hand in hand. A weekend during the holidays is one thing, but if you go six weeks with an increasingly sporadic diet, you can do a tremendous amount of damage. You have worked too long and hard to get here. Don't go backwards.

All of this needs to be infused with a healthy dose of honesty. After a not-so-great weekend of eating, my wife noted that the scale hadn't budged despite her routine exercise during those two days. She started to bemoan that fact, then stopped herself and said, "I haven't done anything this weekend nutritionally to deserve the lower weight so I'm not going to whine about it." The pitfalls are out there. Grab your whip, face the obstacles, and overcome them. Cue the John Williams music—ba ta dump da, ba da daaa . . .

CHAPTER TWELVE KEY POINTS

- 1) Be patient; be prepared.
- 2) Trigger foods are stronger that you are – avoid them, especially in the first few weeks of your diet.
- 3) Plateaus are inevitable but if you stay on target, you will break through!
- 4) Try something new. You're never, ever too old.
- 5) A little hunger won't kill you.
- 6) Find a healthy way to relieve stress.
- 7) You must exercise.

CHAPTER THIRTEEN

THE HEALTH BENEFITS OF GOOD NUTRITION

This is what it is all about. Nutrition, exercise, discipline, fun—it all boils down to improving your health. Many disease states are affected by nutrition, and all of the pages of this text lead to improved physical health and well being. It is true that you can be fat and happy, but you can't be fat and healthy. Now a landmark study in the *New England Journal of Medicine* has shown that you can be fat and exercise or skinny and not exercise, but if you don't incorporate both components of being lean and fit, you are at risk for health problems. Even moderate weight loss can help. Another recent study shows that for people 55 to 75, adding 20 minutes of weightlifting to their aerobic routine can help decrease "metabolic syndrome" by 41%. You are never too old to take good care of yourself. The facts linking obesity and illness will be elucidated in the following pages. Neither Joe nor I have the same gut that your old gym/health/driver's education teacher had, and hopefully you will come away from this chapter with knowledge of some of the dispassionate facts that will spark you to become passionate about taking care of yourself.

Obesity is truly an epidemic in this country, and evidence is now showing that it may eventually replace smoking as the number one cause of preventable death in the United States. Seemingly every study starts with a "gloom and doom" paragraph about the direction our country is heading in regard to expanding our waistlines. A sample platter of these statistics is as follows: currently, more than 60% of U.S. adults are overweight or obese (as defined by having a Body Mass Index, or BMI, greater than 25 and 30 respectively). The prevalence of adult obesity increased an unbelievable 57% between 1991 and 1999. The prevalence of adult (type II) diabetes climbed 765% from 1935 to 1996, and 47 million Americans may have metabolic syndrome in addition to the problems of heart disease, stroke, and arthritis. The statistics are so grim at times we are tempted to simply put our heads in the sand and believe the lie that we can't do anything about it. We can and we must. The numbers reveal this is a war we must win in order to not burden our future generations with unimaginable health care costs.

Obesity can be a chronic condition and should be treated as such. We can stop smoking and drinking, but we can't stop eating. We must make sure what is going into our system is good for us. Let's get with it, and we won't make you put on the ugly gym uniform to do it!

Compare and Contrast

Now before you start getting hives as you flash back to your high-school literature class, this comparison and contrast will be a brief explanation of why certain diets are difficult to maintain over time and why *Metabolic Transformation* is attainable and sustainable. Furthermore, it's not nearly as complicated as comparing and contrasting existentialism between Dostoevsky and Camus. (I frankly can't pronounce Dostoevsky correctly, and I still don't know what the heck a state of existentialism is or if I'd even want to visit there.)

One of the things that give me pause for hope in the health pattern of Americans is that with all the diet controversy a more serious review in both the medical and lay literature is emerging regarding the issue of nutrition. Is it low-fat, low-carb, or just fewer calories that we need to follow? There have been several articles over the last two years that have sought to examine these facts. I have spoken in earlier chapters about the somewhat sneering or condescending challenges brought about by members of the media, and it is time that we answer those challenges. I firmly believe that the American people are smart enough to understand the fundamentals of nutrition and exercise, and want to understand the importance of these things for themselves and their children.

The importance of the macronutrient ranges (The Diet Docs' Rx) is its simplicity that allows you to get a running start on losing weight. However, we want you to become your own nutritionist and ask the question, "Is this something that I really want to put in my body?" (Well, sometimes you may not *want* to eat it, but you may need to.) No longer is it adequate for a physician to tell us that we "need to lose a few pounds." This program gives you an actual plan to accomplish that goal. Why listen to a couple of guys from Indiana? Because if you're serious about weight loss, you need an honest, physiologically sound and practical experience to make it long-term. Leave the bogus promises to others.

Carbs Versus Fat: Round II

The low-carb diet controversy has arguably started people thinking about what we eat. Most importantly, it has challenged the government and the food industry to start to address, in a research-based fashion, how we should properly eat. Carbs of course have become the king, but this new-found nutritional enthusiasm has caused a spillover to look at our old nemesis, dietary fat. The most hopeful thing demonstrated recently is that many manufacturers have pulled trans-fats from their production process. (Remember from chapter six how bad these cats are.) The chemical alteration of these fats leads them to be far more harmful to the arteries. Partially hydrogenated soy, palm, and palm kernel oil used to be staples in snack foods, but now manufacturers are proudly proclaiming "0 grams of trans-fats!" Thanks, guys—it's about freaking time! People have instinctually and correctly believed that the natural dairy fat that's in butter or cheese, along with animal fat, was inherently better for them than any type of chemically altered product. Trans-fats are truly *not* "better living through chemistry." Every family has a story of their 90-year-old grandfather who ate bacon, sausage, and eggs every morning and cooked them all in lard. Mmmm, I can smell it in the frying pan now. However, these folks lived a life of sun-up to sun-down labor that allowed them to burn those calories while improving their musculoskeletal and cardiovascular systems in the process. Furthermore, they ate whole grains full of fiber that naturally helped decrease the body's ability to absorb cholesterol. Today we eat grains that have had all the fiber pounded and bleached out of them, and the only workout we get is the stick shift in the car or the controller on the Playstation.

It is very clear that too much fat is not good for us, and thinking that we can indiscriminately consume any amount of fat just to keep carbs out of our diet is again, not wise. Although the American Heart Association and other organizations may have not gotten everything right with the emphasis on low-fat and higher-carb (I won't say "high- carb" because I honestly don't believe that's what was ever advocated), it has been clearly shown in multiple studies that a diet too high in animal fat increases risks for stroke, heart attack, and certain types of cancer. This does not apply to certain types of plant-based fats or fish oils that have actually shown to be protective. A study in the *Archives of Internal Medicine* showed that one handful of mixed nuts can actually decrease risk of coronary artery disease. Nuts have monounsaturated oils that are thought to help convey protection. The key thing however is "one handful"—which is one ounce, or one serving. Each serving has 15 grams of fat, so don't subscribe to the idea if 1 is good 2 should be better. Getting 30 grams of fat from your snack will likely wreck your fat macronutrient range for the day.

Metabolic Transformation in Action

In June of 2004, I visited my family doctor for my annual physical. I weighed almost 250 pounds, had high blood pressure, and a total cholesterol around 215. The real story on the cholesterol was the triglyceride number. That is the actual fat that cruises through the blood stream. Mine had been very high for several years and the doctor had me on cholesterol-reducing medicine. Now he wanted me to start taking medicine to control my blood pressure. I told the doctor that I have been able to control my blood pressure in the past by losing a little weight. He said "Lose the weight!" I got an e-mail from a friend about his experience with Dr. Joe and the "METABOLIC TRANSFORMATION." Now I had been exercising regularly for several years. I did the weight lifting at the gym and owned my own Aerodyne. I decided to talk to Dr. Joe and was amazed at how easy the nutritional plan was. All you have to do is learn to log what you eat and count protein, carbs, and fat to get the correct balance to metabolize the fat in your body. Exercise is not enough. I read Dr. Joe's book and started eating to live rather than living to eat. Basically, that means only eating what is required for my body to do the work. I immediately saw results in weight loss and realized that I was losing the fat and not the muscle because my weight lifting was improving. In 6 months, I had lost over 50 pounds of fat and my muscle tone became obvious. My cholesterol is in the low-normal range with no medication and my triglycerides are non-existent. My blood pressure and pulse rate are in the very healthy range. This is with nutrition control and no medicine whatsoever. Now, guess what? My family doctor is recommending Dr. Joe to other patients. I'm 49 years old and feel better than I did when I was 30. I can enjoy myself at restaurants and not worry too much on vacations. If I gain a few pounds, I know how to lose the excess in days. It's all about being in control of what goes into your mouth. Dr. Joe is a great encourager and helped me realize that life is worth living to the fullest. If you can do that with nutrition control and reduce the medications – all the better!

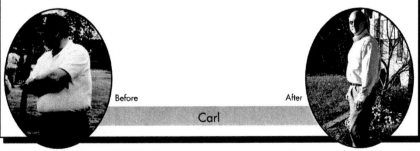

Before — After
Carl

Olive oil has long been known to be protective as well, but again in moderate quantities. Flaxseed oil has been shown to decrease cholesterol, and I have seen one to two tablespoons per day help lower cholesterol in some of my patients. *Metabolic Transformation* allows for fat, but asks you to keep them unsaturated and on the moderate side for health and more rapid weight loss. Fish, especially salmon and tuna, have naturally occurring omega-3 oils that are very good for the arteries and cerebral function. Concern has been raised about mercury levels in fish, and again moderation is the key to getting proper oils without negative effects.

Protein—Our Friend?

You must have lean protein with the emphasis on "lean." Saturated fat is always your enemy to a certain degree if you want to have rock-hard abs. People will tell you, "Oh, you just need to exercise more and your stomach will go away." No it won't. Fat sits in the layer under your skin and *over* your abdominal muscles. You could do 500 crunches a day and if your diet is not in line, you will do an awful lot of work and still not see the results you desire. I know—I've been there. At times I feel like I live there.

Eating protein indiscriminately can produce problems. It is possible to get too much of a good thing. If you eat an excessive amount of protein—calories are calories—insulin can be stimulated, so be careful. Most people, however, do not take in sufficient protein. Adults need about 50 to 70 grams a day for body function, and many of us, especially women, may only get 30 to 40 grams a day. This is part of the reason why in our mid-thirties we start to lose about a half a pound of lean muscle a year. (That and lack of exercise.) You need lean protein combined with exercise to keep your muscles strong.

Carbs, Carbs Everywhere and Not a Drop to Eat

Well now that all those nice Kuebler elves have magically removed the nasty old trans-fats from their products, we should be safe, right? However, several of these foods are still crammed with carbs, and I'm not talking the good kind. The whole idea of "good carbs" and "bad carbs" has been discussed in chapter four. "Good carbs" come from whole grains, certain fruits, and vegetables. Fiber is critically important to help slow carb absorption and further decrease cholesterol absorption. Fiber helps bind cholesterol and limits its uptake. You can think of fiber like a sponge that helps soak up fat and pull it out of your digestive pathway. That's why all those oatmeal boxes have those nice little red "Heart Healthy" logos on them. "Bad carbs" include processed white flour, sugar, high-fructose corn syrup (which is used as a sweetener in just about everything), and certain fruits and vegetables. I am hesitant to label a potato or banana as "bad," but they are much higher in carbs and are absorbed much faster than other produce. The key thing is that faster absorption means more intense insulin spikes. Remember from our previous chapters that insulin is "bad" if you have too much of it circulating because of too many carbs. (Bad hormone, bad! Back to the pancreas where you belong.)

To return to our comparison and contrast: the low-carb diet craze was started to combat the rise in obesity that seemed to center around the increased intake of processed carbs. (Well, that and it was a good marketing niche. I mean, eat bacon, burgers, and butter and lose weight? Sign me up! Not.) Why is processing bad? A study in the *American Journal of Clinical Nutrition* stated that "processing whole grains into white flour actually increases the caloric density greater than 10%, reduces the amount of dietary fiber by 80%, and reduces the amount of dietary protein by 30%." Processing hits us coming and going!

There is no doubt that we take in far too many carbs in our usual diet and it is so darn easy. Slurp down a can of soda—takes a few minutes and there goes 35 to 50 carbs and up to 200 calories. Go to your favorite fast food chain and you may consume over 150 carbs in a single meal. (Yeah, you big boys can have your big toys and your big burgers then go have your big heart attack and face the big medical bill that follows.)

The backlash against carbs was to eat much more of the other two macronutrients (protein and fat) and try to keep carbs to an absolute minimum. However, there are a couple of problems with that logic. Remember, we are never really "cured" of our carb "addiction." Your body will always require a certain amount of carbs to power your central nervous system. Kind of important, eh? You can never, ever be completely carb-free or your body will not function properly, period. You can certainly try to prevent yourself from bingeing on sugar, but you need a certain amount of glucose to power the organ that makes you human and holds all that useless sport and entertainment trivia.

Furthermore, lack of natural fruits, grains, and certain vegetables leads the "low-carbers" to frequently need fiber supplements. Most people aren't really interested in a diet that causes them to spend more time in the bathroom or hundreds of dollars in powdered tree bark. A supplement should be just that—a compliment to an already healthy diet and lifestyle. Natural fiber is crucial for keeping weight down, and in my clinical experience, people would much rather eat their natural fiber than have to mix it up in a glass or take it in a pill. A study by Dr. Simin Liu showed that women who consumed more whole grains not only weighed less but also had a 49% lower risk for weight gain than those that had lower intake. (Now if people refuse to get fiber in their diet, fiber supplements are better than no fiber or the use of laxatives.)

Metabolic Transformation helps limit calories by increasing lean protein to decrease hunger, followed by a moderate amount of healthy carbs and lower fat—a healthy diet that you can follow your whole life. Everyone will have a different spin on how to decrease calories, but you want a diet that you can stick with over time. A systematic review of the efficacy and safety of low-carbohydrate diets presented in the *Journal of the American Medical Association* in April of 2003 came to the following conclusion: "There is insufficient evidence to make recommendations for or against the use of low-carbohydrate diets, particularly among participants older than age 50 years, for use longer than 90 days, or for diets of 20g/day or less of carbohydrates. Among the published studies, participant weight loss while using low-carbohydrate diets was principally associated with decreased caloric intake and increased diet duration but not with reduced carbohydrate content." (Dang, those science geeks are long-winded! But they make a great point.)

We will now talk about some of the health consequences of poor nutrition and finish with how weight loss and proper nutrition can combat some of these diseases. The growing field of nutritional genomics is focusing on the key nutrients in food that actually affects us on a genetic level. Researchers hope to isolate these compounds to help decrease disease risk, including CAD (coronary artery disease), cancer, and Alzheimer's. We will incorporate some of the latest research from this field as we discuss how food can help make us healthier.

Disease States Influenced by Nutrition

The nature of obesity is that it is a chronic relapsing illness that is not cured. I read that in an article and I thought it sounded super cool. I know—I'm a dork. Food is the "agent" that acts on the "host" (that would be you and me) to produce disease. Ideally we would like to use food to *prevent* or *cure* disease rather than be an agent that causes it.

We are quickly discovering that the substances in food not only affect us now, but actually act upon genes (nutritional genomics). Within the next 10 years it may be possible to map those individuals who may be at genetic risk for certain illnesses. (Sounds exciting but would you want to know if you were at higher risk for cancer or Alzheimer's? Would it change the way that you live? Even more importantly, would you want your insurance man to know? What about the person who knows and yet chooses to live an unhealthy lifestyle? An interesting bioethics debate is soon to follow.)

Since we don't have a crystal genetics ball at this point in time, we will talk about some of the known illnesses and how certain foods and weight loss may affect them. One of the most hopeful things that appeared in the media recently was in an article in the January 17th, 2005 issue of *Newsweek*. One of the top researchers in this field was discussing a particular gene variant (Apo E4) that increases risk of diabetes, CAD, and Alzheimer's. The article states that, 15 to 30% of the population may contain at least one copy of this allele . . . but if you stop smoking, give up alcohol, exercise, and eat a diet low in saturated fat 'you can remove *all* genetic predisposition for heart disease that comes with E4." Not just some, but all of it." Food is powerful medicine, but its administration has to be tempered with the realities of everyday living, which is why we are giving you structure with flexibility rather than an exact, precise dose for every single meal or snack for every single second of every single day. (There's only so much anal retentiveness any of us can handle.)

The following obviously cannot be an all inclusive list or expect to provide the detailed information of hundreds of pages of studies and entire chapters from medical textbooks; however, we hope it will highlight the important aspects of how nutrition and exercise can affect our health.

Osteoarthritis, Fibromyalgia, and Chronic Fatigue Syndrome

Osteoarthritis is a very complicated problem, and we still don't have definitive answers for all the causes of premature break down of our joint cartilage. We have seen people who are quite thin their whole lives who have arthritis and some extremely heavy people who don't seem to have any problems with their joints. Exercise and nutrition obviously play a factor in slowing the disease process. The fact of how obesity affects the joints may be a simple lesson in physics: more weight on the joint results in it breaking down faster. Muscles help reduce stress on cartilage, so keeping the muscles strong and the joints mobile further help to reduce pain and degeneration. Decreased intake of calcium, vitamin D, and magnesium may further harm our joints as well as accelerating other physical problems. So where do we get these magic nutrients? Lean dairy, fish, and produce. Glucosamine is a popular supplement that is basically a protein that helps to strengthen and lubricate joints. To learn more about how this supplement got so popular read *The Arthritis Cure*.

A brief aside about vitamin D. Top researchers in the field are becoming distressed at the decrease in the proper production of natural vitamin D (which is produced when our skin is exposed to sunlight) as we spend more time indoors. Dietary vitamin D has declined as we shun dairy and orange juice in our quest for lower carbs. Vitamin D has been shown to have positive affects on breast, prostate, and ovarian cancer as well as rheumatoid arthritis, osteoporosis, and multiple sclerosis. Multiple Sclerosis has long been known to occur more frequently in the northern latitudes, and one of the postulates is that MS is due to decreased sun and consequently decreased vitamin D. Obviously the disease is more complicated than that, but it brings up interesting ideas.

One of the most fit individuals whom I worked with in residency was almost 15 years older than the rest of us, but every day at lunch in addition to his fish and veggies he always had two cartons of skim milk. He could run circles around us. Calcium has been shown to promote weight loss and has long been known to build strong bones and teeth and give you a shiny coat. I know that's why so many doctors play golf—it's for the vitamin D, baby!

Moderate physical exercise is also helpful to maintain joint mobility. If you are leaner and your muscles are stronger, your joints will hurt less! Orthopedic surgeons often will not perform joint replacements, especially total knee replacements, if a patient is substantially overweight. They know that the increased weight will decrease the longevity of the joint and significantly increase the post-operative complication rates. One of the coolest things I saw while on this program were local surgeons referring people to Joe to help lose weight before their operation so that they would have the highest level of success. One such patient received a new knee after losing 50 pounds and then went on to have his other knee replaced after a second 50-pound drop. His surgeon is thrilled to see him riding his mountain bike in his sixth decade of life after many years of being sedentary and pain-ridden.

Exercise, along with physical therapy, has clearly shown to help improve fibromyalgia and chronic fatigue. Fibromyalgia syndrome (FMS) frequently occurs concurrent with arthritis. Often the strain on the muscle which protects the irritated joint will get sore. Proper nutrition to the muscle along with exercise and a treatment modality such as physical therapy, massage, or chiropractic can help decrease the chronic muscle pain without having to take a bunch of pills. Many non-weight bearing or low-impact exercises are now available for people who cannot do the typical walking, jogging, and aerobics. Tai chi, water aerobics, spinning classes, and recumbent exercise bikes—along with the favorite elliptical trainer—are available in almost any gym and are becoming more affordable. Certain insurance companies will, at times, pay for exercise classes, rehabilitation classes, or physical therapy for people with certain diagnoses such as osteoarthritis or cardiac disease. Of course, check with your physician, but these classes may provide an excellent supervised way to get started. Joe recalls a client with the diagnosis FMS who had a history of three whiplash-type injuries. Two minutes on a stationary bike landed her in bed for a week after their first meeting. Light massage therapy, pain meds, and every modality imaginable were a way of life. It took a slow, arduous year of progressive therapeutic exercise combined with a thorough overhaul of her nutrition, but this patient ended up returning to work without pain and now enjoys vigorous workouts.

Chronic fatigue syndrome is poorly understood and has created unbelievable debate in the medical community as to its causes and treatment. B vitamins can certainly help and can be found in whole grains, vegetables, and supplements.

Viruses have also been postulated to play a role, and some factions have wanted the illness renamed "CFIDS" for "chronic fatigue immune deficiency syndrome." (I won't even get into that debate.) Eating right and exercising will improve fatigue and improve your ability to fight disease for a number of reasons. First, decreasing the excessive amount of carbs in your diet will decrease your insulin spikes that make you tired after eating a meal. Second, keeping the sugar down in your bloodstream allows your immune cells to work better. This is one of the reasons why diabetics have trouble fighting disease: the excessive sugar in their blood stream slows proper migration and function of their white blood cells. Although you may not be diabetic, by eating too many carbs and calories, your body's constant clearing of so much sugar will impair your disease-fighting ability. This is part of the reason why people who are overweight and eat poorly seem to have more colds than their skinny-mini, Bowflex-hugging friends.

Lipids, Hypertension, and Cardiovascular Disease

Weight loss, proper nutrition, and exercise all can improve these disease states. Let's examine how obesity can adversely affect these problems.

The result of consuming lipids seems pretty straightforward. If you eat too many, the excess get stuffed into your fat cells, or even worse, they get stuck in your arteries. Pretty basic. True, there is a segment of the population whose lipids may eventually decrease after severely limiting carbs and eating mainly protein and fat instead. However, we have already established how difficult it is to maintain this type of diet for any clinically relevant length of time. For others, low-carb dieting will result in their lipids increasing. It's very difficult when you don't know how your body will react, and this isn't a small gamble! I believe the huge majority of evidence confirms that excessive fat in our diet is not good for us.

We should not advocate a high-carb diet, but neither should we advocate a diet very high in animal fat and cholesterol. Besides increasing our blood lipids, a diet high in animal fat—especially heavily grilled meats—may increase our risk of certain types of cancer such as colorectal. It is critically important to know your entire lipid panel and not just your total cholesterol because a decent total cholesterol may give a false sense of security. I once had a physician friend who had his first heart attack when his cholesterol was 150—well below the recommended 200. However, his HDL was only 15 at the time. Cholesterol panels are broken down into the following: Total Cholesterol (TC), Triglycerides, High-Density Lipoproteins (HDL—the "good" or protective cholesterol), and Low-Density Lipoprotein (LDL—the arch villains of the cholesterol world). It is important to know your entire panel because a poor LDL/HDL ratio can indicate higher risk. Decreasing fat in your diet can help reduce LDL and TC. Decreasing carbs can help lower triglycerides. Finally, exercise can help raise HDL (one of the few things that can raise HDL short of medication), and positively influence the rest of the cholesterol panel. Some vitamins (such as niacin) can decrease triglycerides and raise HDL. "Statin drugs," or HMG Co-A reductase inhibitors, (say that three times fast!) are the primary drugs to lower LDL. They go by many popular names: Lipitor, Pravachol, Zocor, and Crestor. (Now before any of you conspiracy theorists get busy on wondering why I talk about statin drugs, I will say it is because of the following: they save lives. People often don't want to take medicine because they don't want to admit that they are not invincible. I will also make a personal disclosure: I have sold all my individual drug company stock. I have no idea what holdings are in my mutual funds, and I have had family members work in four major pharmaceutical companies so I don't have any preference as to what drug you take. That is between you and your physician.)

If you can't get your lipids under control on this program, then it's probably indicative that you have genetic factors influencing your blood chemistry, and thankfully there are compounds that can prolong your life. Create your own metabolic transformation by faithfully following this program and exercising, and I believe most of you can avoid the medicine chest. But, don't be afraid of medication if you need it. Combined with your exercise and good nutrition, you'll be using the least amount possible.

Newer markers such as VLDL (very low-density lipoprotein), homocysteine levels, and highly-selective, or cardiac C-reactive protein (c-CRP), are being studied as potential early markers for coronary disease. The most important may eventually turn out to be c-CRP because it is a marker for inflammation. Inflammation seems to accelerate the laying down of athrogenic plaques (that gooey stuff inside your arteries that causes them to narrow and increase your risk for a heart attack), and accelerates several illnesses such as Alzheimer's disease, MS, and autoimmune disease. Diet and exercise can positively impact the lipids as well as inflammation. Circulating your blood with exercise helps to pull oxygen and nutrients to all parts of your body so that free radicals and pro-inflammatory substances find it much harder to maintain a foothold.

Hypertension (high blood pressure) is something that can be significantly impacted by weight status. If you are carrying lots of extra adipose (you don't have to cart it out in a little red wagon like Oprah, but you get the picture), your body has to make plenty of extra blood vessels to help keep the fatty tissue alive. Your heart has to pump that much harder to force blood through those miles of extra vessels and your pressure goes up (somewhat of a simplistic explanation, but that's what it boils down to). Shrink the fat, and you decrease the strain on your pump.

Furthermore, if you are eating a healthy diet, you will not be eating a lot of processed food or things with a lot of extra salt. It is true that salt may not have a lot of bearing on certain people with hypertension, but there is certainly a percentage of the population with hypertension, edema (swelling), and CHF (congestive heart failure) who do experience increased blood pressure with higher sodium intake. If you have high blood pressure, take it easy on the salt. People often mistakenly think that since they aren't using the salt shaker that they aren't getting much salt in their diet. You must read labels and pay attention to sodium content if you have these types of problems. Certain soups, processed foods, and snacks may have significant levels of sodium in them. I have seen people wind up in the hospital with a flare-up of their congestive heart failure if they are careless with the sodium in their foods. People will also eat pretzels knowing that they were low-fat and pat themselves on the back about avoiding the high-fat chips (which is good), but not realizing how much sodium they are putting away with their Mister Saltys.

Remember, you are on your way to becoming your own nutritionist! Good health may involve not only knowing proteins, carbs, and fat, but also sodium, potassium, and caffeine content if you are at risk. Reducing hypertension through proper diet and exercise helps decrease the acceleration of atherosclerosis of the arteries and ultimately coronary disease. Wonder why your doctor is always on you to keep your weight and your blood pressure down? Because he knows that all of those things go hand in hand to slow the buildup of plaque in the arteries.

In addition to eating less fat and cholesterol and increasing exercise, certain foods—including fish oil, walnuts, flaxseed oil, and our old friend broccoli—will help decrease lipids and cardiovascular risk. To return to our discussion of nutritional genomics, broccoli has been shown to influence the gene GST, which helps produce the body's master antioxidant, glutathione. This decreases cancer risk and helps keep arteries healthy. Antioxidants help fight free radicals produced in the body that may lead to inflammation or certain types of cancers. And as we've already discussed, no one wants inflamed (or even somewhat incensed or indignant) arteries in their body.

Cancer

Nothing will strike fear in the heart of an otherwise healthy person than the word "cancer." This is such a loaded subject that I almost considered not even including it. However, I do think that we need to make some judicious comments about the subject. I don't want anyone to think that if someone is overweight that they "gave" themselves cancer or that it is their "fault." This disease is far too complex to give such a glib answer. Also, thin people—including world class athletes—get cancer too as we've witnessed in the wonderful triumph of Lance Armstrong. (One of the drugs that helped cure him came from tree bark.) Furthermore, I would not want people to abandon proven scientific treatment to rely simply on nutrition. However, several links between obesity and cancer have been drawn and confirmed. Increased weight can have negative effects on certain tumors. Good nutrition can positively affect your treatment whereas poor nutrition can increase risk factors. One recent study showed that eating french fries just twice a week increased the risk of breast cancer 27 times! Soybeans affect 123 genes involved in prostate cancer and help to block tumor formation. We've already talked about broccoli and vitamin D. As our friends in research continue to pound away, stay tuned on how the food you put into your body every day can help decrease your risk of cancer. There are already volumes of comprehensive books detailing the micronutritional content of certain foods and their positive effects on cancer prevention and their curative properties. Guess what foods make up, oh, about 99.9% of this list? Fruits and vegetables.

Diabetes type II

Diabetes mellitus type II (DM II) and metabolic syndrome are two of the diseases that are significantly affected by our weight. Approximately 90% of diabetes is non-insulin dependent, or diabetes type II (also known as adult onset diabetes). Type I (insulin-dependent) will not be discussed here. Our genetics obviously influence our ability to get these diseases, but the good news according to the textbooks and recent studies is that even a moderate weight loss (as little as 10 pounds) may significantly decrease the risk of the disease and limit also its impact on your health. As we discussed earlier, exercise will improve our cardiovascular risk, assist in losing body fat, and reduce our BMI (body mass index), but it will also decrease our diabetes risk. Exercise will also positively influence DM, but not as much as if incorporated with weight loss.

The epidemiology of diabetes makes it critical that we continue to try to defeat this disease. Our rapidly increasing waistlines mean rapid increases in DM II cases. Conservative studies show that diabetes accounts for about 15% of health care costs in the U.S. and its consequences can be tragically debilitating. According to the *Cecil Textbook of Medicine*: "It is the leading cause of blindness, end-stage renal disease, and non-traumatic limb amputations." Furthermore, it increases cardiovascular complications, peripheral vascular disease, and neuropathy, a very painful, chronic burning condition in the extremities. The scary thing is that the symptoms for diabetes such as excessive thirst, excessive urination, weight loss, blurred vision, and dizziness may be subtle and ignored for a long time. Some texts and studies speculate that there may be one undiagnosed diabetic for every known case. This is one disease for which you really need to be tested if you are overweight, especially around your middle, or if there is a family history. Even better, keeping your weight down throughout your life will significantly reduce your risk. Diabetes is a combination of decreased insulin secretion and increased insulin resistance. Insulin resistance is clearly linked to increasing obesity. In other words, a life of eating too many carbohydrates, causing too much insulin to be secreted, will cause your whole body to become desensitized.

Diet and weight loss combined is truly the key. I often tell my patients that treating diabetes is like a triangle: the three parts of the triangle are diet, physical activity, and medication. If you neglect any one part of that triangle, the other two parts have to be stretched to make up for that deficiency. Diet and activity are within your control and are the keys to help manage this disease. Even if you have to start taking medicine, diet and exercise should be paramount. Keeping fat and carbs lower and lean protein higher is important. Weight reduction will help keep blood glucose in check. Exercise will keep your body using blood sugar as energy, thus keeping overall blood sugar lower. Even though you may not be able to achieve a total cure, keeping these two parts of the triangle under control may delay the need for medication or result in a decreased dose. In disease states such as hypertension, diabetes, and hyperlipidemia, you must keep your sugar, lipids, and blood pressure under the tightest control for the longest time possible. Most of the damage caused by these illnesses is cumulative over time. Though you may be able to eliminate or avoid a lot of medication, which is our goal, you need to start your medicine if your doctor prescribes it, and use it until he says otherwise. There is no sense having a disease, going to your doctor, and then just halfway controlling it. Your doctor would love nothing more than if you were an active participant—a teammate—to increase the quality and length of your life. Work with your physician if you want to have the greatest, healthiest life span possible.

Alzheimer's

Alzheimer's pathophysiology is still not completely understood and older Americans are rightly fearful of the words "Alzheimer's disease." Curry powder contains turmeric, which has been shown to suppress genes that increase inflammation. Inflammation has been implicated in not only heart disease and colon cancer but Alzheimer's as well. India has one of the lowest incidences of Alzheimer's in the world, and turmeric is thought to play a role in that low occurrence. Exercise and anti-inflammatories may positively affect this disease. Mental activity, such as reading and crossword puzzles, "exercises" your brain and can slow even normal neurological aging. Physical exercise increases the blood flow that carries healthy nutrition directly to the brain. As we've already stressed, a diet low in sugar and fat causes less inflammation than a diet high in sugar and fat. It's more complicated than this, but there is cause for optimism.

The Granddaddy of them All: Metabolic Syndrome

So what is this thing called "metabolic syndrome" and why should we care? First of all, do not get "metabolic syndrome" confused with *Metabolic Transformation*! Okay, everyone clear on that one?! We should care because metabolic syndrome is one of the fastest growing disease states in the United States. This illness has gone by a number of names in the past, such as syndrome X, dysmetabolic syndrome, or insulin resistance syndrome. This condition includes abdominal obesity, abnormal lipids, elevated blood pressure, insulin resistance, a prothrombotic state (making you more prone to blood clots), and a proinflammatory state (remember how important we have said inflammation is? I know, that horse died a paragraph or two ago).

If you get metabolic syndrome, you will be on the fast track to heart disease and diabetes. How fast, you ask? I have seen patients with metabolic syndrome as young as their late 30's and early 40's with full-blown heart disease that required intervention such as angioplasty or even open heart surgery. A recent study from the *Third National Health and Nutrition Examination Survey (NHANES III)* stated that 47 million Americans have metabolic syndrome. Good grief, Charlie Brown, that's 24% of the U.S. population! Have you ever seen the bill for a cardiac cath? On an even more serious note, one in four heart attacks result in death. That's right folks, death. No little guys with the paddles, no family members patting your hand in the ICU. Dead, gone, that's it. It's not well-publicized, but that's a fact, Jack.

So, how is this disease state defined? For men, an abdominal waist circumference greater than 40 inches; and for women, greater than 35 inches starts your membership to this dubious club. (Run get that tape measure! It doesn't mean the smallest pair of jeans you can squeeze yourself into before you pass out from asphyxia.) Further criteria include triglycerides > 150; HDL < 40 for men and < 50 for women; blood pressure > 130/85, and finally, fasting glucose > 110. People who have any three of the five criteria qualify as having metabolic syndrome. Obesity, lack of activity, and genetic factors all contribute to the illness, and excessive body fat and inactivity accelerate the expression of those genes.

We can't trade our genes in for a new set just yet. As stated in a recent publication regarding metabolic syndrome, "The greatest potential of benefit from management of metabolic syndrome lies in reversing its root causes: overweight/obesity and physical inactivity." Why is obesity important? Let's return to that same publication. "Abdominal/visceral adiposity is associated with an increased release of free fatty acids into the portal blood, which, in turn, leads to hepatic overproduction of triglycerides and decreased synthesis of high-density lipoprotein cholesterol, both characteristic of metabolic syndrome." In other words, having a fat tummy releases toxins in your system and decreases your body's ability to produce the good stuff to fight those toxins. (Now that sounds a little nicer than that mean old scientific jargon, doesn't it?)

So the long and the short of it is that if we are carrying a lot of weight in our abdomen and chest, that fatty tissue is releasing substances that will harm us. This is why people with the "apple" shape rather than the "pear" shape need to get to their physicians and not just their plastic surgeons. Increased weight increases insulin resistance, which in turn will increase blood sugar, blood pressure, and negative lipid profiles. Since the receptors on the tissues are not as sensitive, your body has to pump out more and more insulin to get the same response. We have talked earlier about how excessive insulin is an enemy, and this condition quickly turns into a viscous cycle of insulin resistance, increased insulin, weight gain, and then further insulin release! This will eventually lead to type II diabetes and then all the increased problems that go along with that. Hypertension is at least twice as common in patients with type II diabetes as it is in patients without the disease. Furthermore, patients with hypertension are twice as likely to develop diabetes over a four-to-five year period. Hypertension then accelerates the complications of diabetes, especially stroke, kidney disease, and diabetic eye disease.

So what can we do to stop the slide? Um, how 'bout diet and exercise. And it doesn't matter what age you are. One 5,000-person study showed that intentional weight loss in people with this disease decreased mortality by 25%. Another recent study showed that "104 adults aged 55 to 75 reduced their rate of metabolic syndrome by 41% after 6 months by adding 20 minutes of weightlifting to their aerobic routine." I see plenty of older people at the gym hitting the machines, and they are doing it and doing it well. Now they may not have abs like LL Cool J, and you can sometimes see the big ol' bodybuilders getting a little annoyed that granny is monopolizing their machine. However, studies like these prove that older people can improve their health, so go drink a protein shake, Sonny, and come back in a few minutes. As I stated earlier, dropping as few as 10 pounds and reducing blood pressure by 10 points can decrease the damage from these diseases. Indeed, some studies have gone so far as to indicate that if we achieved optimal control over the risk factors, the disease may be reduced by 80%! Food (and exercise) for thought.

Nutritional Genomics; Why Should We Care about Another Two-Dollar Word?

This is something very interesting to keep a close watch on. We have discussed some of the exciting discoveries above. Ever since Dr. Sears talked about "eicosanoids," the friendly little quarks of the nutritional world, a bridge between science and the layman's understanding of nutrition has developed. I believe this field holds the most promise as they isolate the chemicals in food and the particular genes that they act on. This will help finally take a bit of the nebulous nature out of nutrition and start to pin down some hardcore pathways that could help benefit our bodies. The next vexing question, however, is: how much should we eat of certain things? Would a pound of broccoli a day be enough to cut down our disease risks, and if that's what it takes, do you want to be the one to sit next to that person on the bus?

Fitness Versus Fatness—Let's End this Debate, Shall We?

Two key articles were presented in the *New England Journal of Medicine* and the *Journal of the American Medical Association* (JAMA) at the end of 2004. To summarize, it appears that physical inactivity is the main risk factor for cardiovascular disease and BMI is the main risk factor for diabetes. They each influence the other to a certain degree, but this is the direction these studies were pointing. This research was in women, so stand in line, guys. We do know that there will probably be a correlation in men (how strong that correlation is remains to be seen). The guy in the Bowflex commercial is calling out Jared about eating sandwiches. I love Jared, and he and Subway have raised awareness extensively in the fast food sector. (If you want to be really, really scared then skip *Friday the 13th XXIX* and get Morgan Spurlock's brave and brilliant *Super Size Me*. You may never go back in the water with fast food again.) You know this doesn't have to be like the North and the South with the damn Yankees of diet and the southern boys of exercise. You need both. Don't think that if you haven't achieved six-pack abs yet that you are a failure either. I often run into the rationalization that people will say, "Hey, I exercise; I can eat what I want," or "I eat healthy; I don't need to exercise." As we discussed above, you must have *both* for total health.

Health Doesn't Care

Now, let's be very, very clear about something. No one needs to be "prejudiced" against people who are overweight. There is no more reason to be prejudiced against them than another person of a different race, nationality, religion, etc. All people deserve to be loved and respected. We don't need to be any more prejudiced against an overweight person than we do against someone with diabetes, heart disease, or any other disease state. But we do need to acknowledge that being overweight even moderately will put us at higher risk for significant health problems. Study after study has shown us that. We all know of the person who smoked too much, drank too much, or ate too much and lived to be 100. But I can tell you story after story of people who were substantially overweight, which cost them their lives in their 30's and 40's. And then there are all the days of using canes, walkers, wheel chairs, oxygen tanks, hospital beds, and the general debility that may accompany serious weight problems. We have also discussed how you can be thin, and if you are not exercising and not putting proper fuel in your body, you are missing out on optimal health as well.

We should love ourselves, but we should love ourselves enough to take care of ourselves. For you see, health doesn't care. Health doesn't care if your father or mother was mean or cruel to you growing up. Health doesn't care that you hate your job or that life is stressful. It doesn't care; it just is what it is.

You can love yourself fat or thin and you can pretty well hate yourself fat or thin. Try getting out of denial at both extremes, getting the help that you need physically and emotionally, and try loving yourself enough to get healthy. I have known my wife since high school, which covers a 155- to 230-pound weight swing and all spaces in between. I have always felt loved no matter what I weighed. "Love" was never the issue. But as my blood pressure reached 170/105, she was gravely concerned about my health. I didn't "love" myself enough to care about the imminent risks to my own well being, and that is the key. Until I cared about the *reality* of my declining physical health, only then could I take the steps to care for myself.

Now you say, "But Dr. Uloth, I may be 30, 40, or 50 pounds overweight, but I don't smoke or drink and my blood pressure and lipids are good. I exercise three or four days a week. What's your problem?" The problem is the evidence from the studies cited above. The evidence is unblinking and unflinching and comes with no malice or prejudice. You may be fine now, but you have significantly increased your risk of future problems. I sincerely believe that my years of poor eating habits along with my excessive weight have shortened my life span. I can do everything now in my power to reverse that trend, but there is some damage that has been done and I cannot take it back. That doesn't mean that I'm not going to try or that I'm going to say, "What the heck," and go with the flow. I want to stick around for my wife and my children and the people I care for on a day-to-day basis. Dying versus living healthy—compare and contrast that for a while.

CHAPTER THIRTEEN KEY POINTS

▶ 1) Good nutrition is critical for good health. Duh.

▶ 2) Nutrition can affect you even at the genetic level. (Now that's heavy duty.)

▶ 3) Weight affects your diabetes risk. Exercise can affect your cardiovascular risk. And your knee bone connects to your hip bone…

▶ 4) Remember: health doesn't care, so you should.

CHAPTER FOURTEEN

KEEP IT OFF FOREVER!

There would be nothing more disheartening than to gain back a significant portion of the weight you lost once you've worked so hard for so long. You may already know exactly what I'm talking about from past experience. You can stop this pattern if you take this transition seriously.

Some of the blame for this misfortune lies, again, at the foot of physiology. The habits created when dieting and the excitement of success held you to your previous diet. However, if that plan included a severe decrease in carbohydrates or insufficient calories, your metabolic rate may have suffered significantly. Once a higher food intake is reestablished, you may have regained body fat rapidly until your metabolic rate rebounded. By then, it was too late. That is the danger of a very low-calorie or low-carb diet.

A second reason for failure, and often in conjunction with the first, is letting your guard down and not adjusting your food properly. If you were to plow through a few days of really high-carb intake, especially the typical binge or "celebration" foods, it is very hard to recover. The wildly fluctuating blood sugar will spin you into levels of hunger you aren't used to. Before you know it, you're eating an incredible amount of carbohydrates and converting a large portion of them into body fat again. This is the exact cycle you bought this book to avoid.

Once you have reached your goal, you have to bring your food intake up to a maintenance level where you will no longer be losing, but, of course, not gaining. You will not have to raise your protein levels; they have already been set to give you an ideal amount. Your fat and carbohydrates may be raised in tandem but not necessarily in equal amounts. You may find that 10 to 15 extra grams of fat and 25 grams of carbs will provide enough energy and calories as the first step toward raising your food intake to a maintenance level. This may slow your rate of loss, but not stop it completely. Take another step upward, and then another.

Many important things will happen if you make this process incremental. First, your blood chemistry will remain more stable and you'll be less likely to experience binge-causing hunger due to the increase in carbohydrates. Second, you'll slowly rebuild any decreases in your metabolic rate that may have occurred due to the length of your diet. This will ensure that you won't regain body fat at all. As a matter of fact, you'll find you have to slowly keep adding more food to not lose weight! The amount of carbohydrates and fat that you add is entirely up to you, but keep several health and behavioral points in mind.

You still want to adhere to the same health-building habits that you created along the way. Keep good fats in your diet and keep saturated fats low. Stick with low-glycemic index carbs as much as you can (for all the reasons you dieted with them). If you can maintain most of these principles, your increase in food will leave you with high energy, stability, and controlled weight. Experiment with different levels of carbohydrates and fat at your decided maintenance level of food. You may find that you feel and "operate" better with one macronutrient raised disproportionately to the other. This has to do with metabolic body type. An insulin-sensitive person may get hungrier on a higher level of carbs and tend to gain weight back. However, with carbs remaining a little lower and fat increasing, the same person may have no hunger, high energy, and no weight gain. A person fortunate enough to have a high metabolism tends to be an "ectomorph" and be able to consume a higher percentage of calories from carbs without weight gain. Beware, though, despite being able to get away with more carbs, an ectomorph can still gain weight.

One last point: as you transition into maintenance, you are leaving a dieting level of food that includes less carbs than your body needs for energy. As you increase your food, you will be refilling your liver and muscles with a higher amount of glycogen. Glycogen attracts and holds water. You will undoubtedly gain a couple of pounds due to that fact just as the first couple of lost pounds were water. Don't be alarmed; this is normal hydration and a normal level of carbohydrates stored in your body. You just want to make sure you don't gain more than a couple pounds back once you've hit your lowest weight. Your body fat level won't be affected; the weight will be just water and glycogen. This is another reason to keep your upward changes slow and incremental. You don't want to fret over water gain, but you also don't want to be deceived into thinking that you're gaining just water when it may be fat.

So, there you have it. If patiently and scientifically handled, the transition into maintenance can be smooth and successful. Instead of regain, you can have an increasing level of energy, an increasing metabolic rate, and control of your weight. That, after all, is our goal for you.

EPILOGUE

A DIET DOC—THREE YEARS LATER

By the time this book is released and has made it into your hot little hands, it will have been almost three years since I walked into Joe's office on January 29, 2004. Talk about a moment that can change your life! It doesn't rank up there with my wedding day, the birth of my children, graduation from medical school, or that time I hit three home runs in one game in the eighth grade (sorry Joe). However, I know where I would have wound up if I hadn't changed my lifestyle. Surveys have shown that physicians have one of the lowest life spans for professionals at only 58 years of age. For many, they're dead before they even reach retirement. I didn't want to end up a statistic. Caring for others on a daily basis is unbelievably rewarding and unbelievably draining at the same time (just ask my wife). Fortunately, I know now that you can indeed care for others and care for yourself. It has not been easy. The first holidays after my weight loss were very difficult, shoulder and knee injuries have slowed my training and will probably result in eventual surgery, and sometimes life is just hard and stressful. But you know what? Now I have the knowledge I need to get myself back on track and stay there. I don't stumble around in the dark breathing more rapidly as the anxiety slowly but steadily mounts. Am I going to fail again? Is 230 pounds just around the corner? The fear of not knowing where to turn or what to do is gone. The fear has been replaced with understanding. I feel empowered and I am filled with gratitude for discovering this program. I have benefited, my patients have benefited, and now hopefully you will benefit as well. I won't see 230, or even 200 for that matter, ever again. Be gone little blinking red lights! Be gone foul harbingers of my own doom! I guess I could have taken the batteries out that first day, but that's not the point. I am now my own nutritionist. I am busy living, and I hope you will be too. Good luck and God bless.

BIBLIOGRAPHY

Abbasi, F., et al. 2000. "High carbohydrate diets, triglyceride rich lipoproteins, and coronary heart disease risk." *American Journal of Cardiology* 85:45-48.

Acheson, K.J., et al. 1984. "Nutritional influences on lipogenesis and thermogenesis after a carbohydrate meal." *American Journal of Physiology* 246:E62-E70.

Agus, M.S.D., et al. 2000. "Dietary composition and physiologic adaptations to energy restriction." *American Journal of Clinical Nutrition* 71:901-7.

Ascherio, A., and W.C. Willet. 1997. "Health effects of transfatty acids." *American Journal of Clinical Nutrition* 66:1006S-1010S.

Atkins, R.C. 2002. *Dr. Atkins' New Diet Revolution*. Avon, New York, NY.

Baba, N.H., et al. 1999. "High protein versus high carbohydrate hypoenergetic diet for the treatment of obese hyperinsulinemic subjects." *International Journal of Obesity* 11:1202-1206.

Brand-Miller, J.C. et al. 2002. "Glycemic index and obesity." *American Journal of Clinical Nutrition* 76:281S-285S.

Brand-Miller, J., et al. 2003. *The New Glucose Revolution*. Marlowe and Company, New York, NY.

Bravata, D.M., L. Sanders, J. Huang, et al. 2003. "Efficacy and safety of low-carbohydrate diets: a systematic review." *Journal of the American Medical Association* 289;14:1837-1850.

Bray, G.A. 1969. "Effect of caloric restrictions on energy expenditure in obese patients." *Lancet* 2:397-8.

Bray, G.A. 2003. "Low-carbohydrate diets and realities of weight loss." *Journal of the American Medical Association* 289;14:1853-1855.

Brody, T. 1999. *Nutritional Biochemistry*, Second ed. Academic Press, San Diego, CA.

Brownell, K.D., M.R.C. Greenwood, E. Stellar, and E.E. Shrager. 1986. "The effects of repeated cycles of weight loss and regain in rats." *Physiology Behavior* 38:459-64.

Campfield, L., F. Smith, and P. Burn. 1998. "Strategies and potential molecular targets for obesity treatment." *Science* 280:1383-1387.

Carlola, R., J.P. Harley, and C.R. Noback. 1990. *Human Anatomy and Physiology*. McGraw-Hill, New York, NY.

Chinachoti, P. 1995. "Carbohydrates: Functionality in foods." *American Journal of Clinical Nutrition* 61:922S-929S.

Clark, L.T., K.C. Ferdinand, and D.P. Ferdinand. 2003. *Contemporary Management of the Metabolic Syndrome*. McMahon Publishing Group, New York, NY.

Crapo, P.A. 1985. "Simple versus complex carbohydrate use in the diabetic diet." *Annual Review of Nutrition* 5:95-114.

Daly, M.E. et al. 1997. "Dietary carbohydrate and insulin sensitivity: A review of the evidence and clinical implications." *American Journal of Clinical Nutrition* 66:1072-1085.

Depres, J.P., et al. 1996. "Hyperinsulinemia as an independent risk factor for ischemic heart disease." *New England Journal of Medicine* 334:952-957.

Dune, L.J. 1990. *Nutrition Almanac*, 3rd ed. McGraw-Hill, New York, NY.

Eades, M.R. and M.D. Eades. 1996. *Protein Power*. Bantam Books, New York, NY.

Ely, D.L. 1997. "Overview of dietary sodium effects on and interactions with cardiovascular and neuroendocrine functions." *American Journal of Clinical Nutrition* 65:594S-605S.

Erikson, R.H. and Y.S. Kim. 1990. "Digestion and absorption of dietary protein." *Annual Review of Medicine* 41:133-139.

Felig, P., et al. 1970. "Amino acid metabolism in the regulation of gluconeogenesis in man." *American Journal of Clinical Nutrition* 23:986-992.

Felig, P., J.D. Baxter, and L.A. Frohman. 1995. *Endocrinology and Metabolism*, 3rd ed. McGraw-Hill, New York, NY.

Figlewicz, D.P., et al. 1996. "Endocrine regulation of food intake and body weight." *Journal of Laboratory and Clinical Medicine* 127:328-332.

Fisler, J.S., et al. 1982. "Nitrogen economy during very low calorie reducing diets." *American Journal of Clinical Nutrition* 35:471-486.

Flegal, K.M., B.I. Graubard, D.F. Williamson, and M.H. Gail. 2005. "Excess deaths associated with underweight, overweight, and obesity." *Journal of the American Medical Association* 293;15:1861-68.

Ford, E.S., and S.Liu. 2001. "Glycemic index and serum high-density-lipoprotein cholesterol concentration among US adults." *Archives of Internal Medicine* 161:572-48.

Fordslund, A.H., et al. 1999. "Effect of protein intake and physical activity on twenty-four hour pattern and rate of micronutrient utilization." *American Physiology Society* E964-E976.

Foster-Powell, K., J.C. Brand-Miller, S.H.A. Holt. 2002. "International table of glycemic index and glycemic load values: 2002." *American Journal of Clinical Nutrition* 76:5-56.

Fraser, G.E., J. Sabate, W.L. Beeson, and T.M. Strahan. 1992. "A Possible Protective Effect of Nutrition Consumption on Risk of Coronary Heart Disease—The Adventist Health Study." *Archives of Internal Medicine* 152:1416-1424.

Friedman, H.I. and B. Nylund. 1980. "Intestinal fat digestion, absorption, and transport." *American Journal of Clinical Nutrition* 33:1108-1139.

Frost, G. and A. Dornhorst. 2000. "The relevance of the glycemic index to our understanding of dietary carbohydrates." *Diabetic Medicine* 17:336-45

Fushiki, T., et al. 1989. "Changes in glucose transporters in muscle in response to glucose." *American Journal of Physiology* 256:E580-E587.

Golay, A., et al. 1996. "Weight loss with low or high carbohydrate diet?" *International Journal of Obesity and Related Metabolic Disorders* 20:1067-1072.

Goldman, L. and J.C. Bennett. 2000. *Cecil Textbook of Medicine* 21st ed. Saunders, Philadelphia, PA.

Gottfried, S.S. 1993. *Biology Today.* Mosby, St. Louis, MO.

Groff, J.L. and S.S. Gropper. 2000. *Advanced Nutrition and Human Metabolism.* Wadsworth Thomson Learning, Stamford, CT.

Gross, L.S., E.S. Ford, and S. Liu. 2004. "Increased consumption of refined carbohydrates and the epidemic of type 2 diabetes in the United States:an ecologic assessment." American *Journal of Clinical Nutrition*.79:774-9.

Holloszy, J. and W. Kohrt. 1996. "Regulation of carbohydrate and fat metabolism during and after exercise." *Annual Review of Nutrition* 16:121-138.

Holman, R.T. 1988. "George O. Burr and the discovery of essential fatty acids." *Journal of Nutrition* 118:535-540.

Hu, F.B., W.C. Willett, T. Li, et al. 2004. "Adiposity as compared with physical activity in predicting mortality among women." *New England Journal of Medicine* 351:2694-703.

Hudgins, L., et al. 2000. "Relationship between carbohydrate induced hypertriglyceridemia and fatty acid synthesis in lean and obese subjects." *Journal of Lipid Research* 41:595-604.

Jenkins, D.J., C.W. Kendall, A. Marchie, and L.S. Augustin. 2004. "Too much sugar, too much carbohydrate, or just too much?" *American Journal of Clinical Nutriton* 79:711-2.

Leaf, A. and P.C. Weber. 1988. "Cardiovascular effects of n-3 fatty acids." *New England Journal of Medicine* 318:549-557.

Leeds, A.R. 2002. "Glycemic index and heart disease." *American Journal of Clinical Nutrition* 76:286S-289S.

Leibel, R.L., M. Rosenbaum, and J. Hirsch. 1995. "Changes in energy expenditure resulting from altered body weight." *New England Journal of Medicine* 332:621-628.

Leibowitz, S.F. 1992. "Neurochemical-neuroendocrine systems in the brain controlling macronutrient intake and metabolism." *Trends in Neuroscience* 15:491-497.

Liu, Simmin, W.C. Willett, J.E. Manson, et al. 2003. Relation between changes in intakes in dietary fiber and grain products and changes in weight and development of obesity among middle aged women." American Journal of Clinical Nutrition 78:920-7.

Jacobson, M.F. and J. Hurley. 2002. *Restaurant Confidential.* Workman Publishing, New York, NY.

McArdle, W.D., F.I. Katch, and V.L. Katch. 1991. *Exercise Physiology: Energy, Nutrition, and Human Performance,* Third ed. Lea and Febiger, Malvern, PA.

Millward, D.J. 1998. "Metabolic demands for amino acids and the human dietary requirement." *Journal of Nutrition* 2563S-2576S.

Morris, K., et al. 1999. "Glycemic index, cardiovascular disease, and obesity." *Nutrition Reviews* 57:273-276.

Murray, M.T. and J. Beutler. 1996. *Understanding Fats and Oils.* Progressive Health Publishing, Encinitas, CA.

Nelson, J.K., et al. 1994. *Mayo Clinic Diet Manual: A Handbook of Nutrition Practices,* Seventh ed. Mosby, St. Louis, MO.

Netzer, C.T. 2003. *The Complete Book of Food Counts.* Dell Publishing, New York, NY.

Nicholl, C.G., J.M. Polak, and S.R. Bloom. 1985. "The hormonal regulation of food intake, digestion, and absorption." *Annual Review of Nutrition* 5:213-239.

Nobels, F., et al. 1989. "Weight reduction with a high protein, low carbohydrate, caloric restricted diet: Effects on blood pressure, glucose, and insulin levels." *Netherlands Journal of Medicine* 35:295-302.

Pieke., B., et al. 2000. "Treatment of hypertriglyceridemia by two diets rich either in unsaturated fatty acids or in carbohydrates: Effects on lipoprotein subclasses, lipolytic enzymes, lipid transfer proteins, insulin, and leptin. *International Journal of Obesity* 24:1286-1296.

Pilkis, S.J., et al. 1988. "Hormonal regulation of hepatic gluconeogenesis and glycolysis." *Annual Review of Biochemistry* 57:755-783.

Rabast, U., J. Schonborn, and H. Kasper. 1979. "Dietetic treatment of obesity with low—and high-carbohydrate diets: comparative studies and clinical results." *International Journal of Obesity* 3(3):201-11.

Reed, W.D., et al. 1984. "The effects of insulin and glucagons on ketone-body turnover." *Biochemistry* 221:439-444.

Reeds, P.J. and T.W. Hutchens. 1994. "Protein requirements: From nitrogen balance to functional impact." *Journal of Nutrition* 1754S-1963-S.

Richter, E.A., T. Ploug, and H. Galbo. 1985. "Increased muscle glucose uptake after exercise." *Diabetes* 34:1041-1048.

Scriver, C.R., et al. 1985. "Normal plasma amino acid values in adults: The influence of some common physiological variables." *Metabolism* 34:868-873.

Sears, B. and B. Lawren. 1995. *Enter the Zone.* Harper Collins, New York, NY.

Sims, E.A. 1974. "Studies in human hyperphagia." *Treatment and Management of Obesity.* New York, Harper and Row.

Souba, W.W., R.J. Smith, and D.W. Wilmore. 1985. "Glutamine Metabolism by the intestinal tract." *Journal of Parenteral Enteral Nutrition* 9:608-617.

Stewart, K.J., A.C. Bacher, K. Turner, et al. 2005. "Exercise and Risk Factors Associated with Metabolic Syndrome in Older Adults." *American Journal of Preventative Medicine* 28(1):9-18.

Stordy, B.J., et al. 1977. "Weight gain, thermic effects of glucose and resting metabolic rate during recovery from anorexia nervosa." *American Journal of Clinical Nutrition* 30:138.

The Life Application Study Bible NIV translation.1991. Tyndale and Zondervan. Tyndale House Publishers, Wheaton, IL.

Thorne, A. and J. Wahren. 1989. "Diet-induced thermogenesis in well-trained subjects." *Clinical Physiology* 0:295-305.

Traxinger, R.R. and S. Marshall. 1989. "Role of amino acids in modulating glucose-induced desensitization of the glucose transport system." *Journal of Biological Chemistry* 264:20910-20916.

Underwood, A. and J. Adler. Jan. 17, 2005 "Diet and genes." *Newsweek* 40-8.

Weinstein, A.R., H.P. Sesso, I.M. Lee., et al. 2004. "Relationship of physical activity versus body mass index with type II diabetes in women." *Journal of the American Medical Association* 292;10:1188-9.

Wessel, T.R., C.B. Arant, M.B. Olson, et al. 2004. "Relationship of physical fitness versus body mass index with coronary artery disease and cardiovascular events in women." *Journal of the American Medical Association* 292;10:1179-87.

Westphal, S.A., M.C. Gannon, and F.Q. Nutrall. 1990. "Metabolic response to glucose ingested with various amounts of protein." *American Journal of Clinical Nutrition* 62:267-272.

Whitney, E.N. and S.R. Rolfes. 1996. *Understanding Nutrition*, Seventh ed. West Publishing Company, St. Paul, MN.

Woods, S.C., et al. 1998. "Signals that regulate food intake and energy homeostasis." *Science* 280:1378-1383.

Wolfe, B.M. 1995. "Potential role of raising dietary protein intake for reducing risk of atherosclerosis." *Canadian Journal of Cardiology* 11:127G-131G.

Yamada, T., et al. 1995. *Textbook of Gastroenterology*, Second ed. J.B. Lippincott Company, Philadelphia, PA.

Young, D.B., et al. 1984. "Effects of sodium intake on steady-state potassium excretion." *American Journal of Physiology* 246:F772-F778.

Young, V.R. and J.S. Marchini. 1990. "Mechanisms and nutritional significance of metabolic responses to altered intakes of protein and amino acids, with reference to nutritional adaption in humans." *American Journal of Clinical Nutrition* 51:270-289.

Bill Murphy

- Motivation
- Commitment
- Goals Setting — have them in order of importance
  ↓ vs how are you living your life
- How do you perceive things — be positive
- Visualisation... yourself smell, touch, feel, see
- Have confidence in your ability to succeed
- Always believe like Coach Belichek

- Dream... and aim high don't aim low you come in lower.
- "Why" Ask yourself — write down goals and whys
- Utilize your resources
- Accountability... tell others
- Inspirational quotes...
- Calendar... time frame put it on there

★ Need them

Learn — What type are you,
  Hear something, See something
  Do it

★ How do you learn to change the oil in your car?
  I am a "Do it" person... → (a model's picture)

Do you move towards something or away from something (picture of me)